Herbalism and Natural Remedies for Beginners & Foraging Wild Edible Plants 2-in-1 Compilation

FIELD GUIDE TO OVERCOMING COMMON AILMENTS FROM HOME & IDENTIFYING, HARVESTING, AND PREPARING EDIBLE WILD PLANTS AND HERBS

Small Footprint Press

THIS COLLECTION INCLUDES THE FOLLOWING BOOKS:

The Great Survival Book of Foraging Wild Edible Plants

The Holistic Book of Herbal Medicine & Natural Remedies

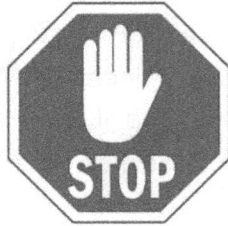

BEFORE YOU START READING, DOWNLOAD YOUR FREE BONUSES!

Scan the QR-code & Access
all the Resources for FREE!

SCAN ME

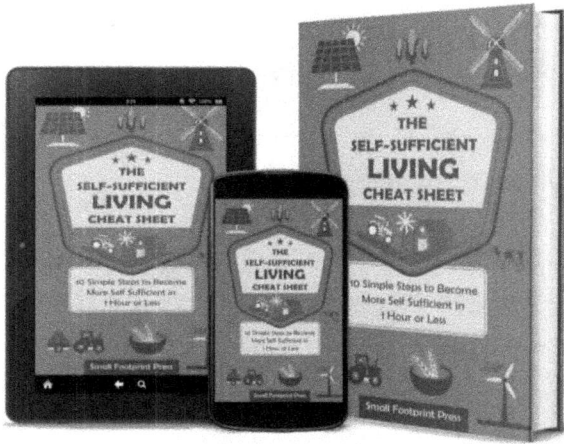

The Self-Sufficient Living Cheat Sheet

10 Simple Steps to Become More Self-Sufficient in 1 Hour or Less

How to restore balance to the environment around you... even if you live in a tiny apartment in the city.

Discover:

- **How to increase your income** by selling "useless" household items

- The environmentally friendly way to replace your car — invest in THIS special vehicle to **eliminate your carbon footprint**

- The secret ingredient to **turning your backyard into a thriving garden**

- 17+ different types of food scraps and 'waste' that you can use to feed your garden

- How to drastically **cut down on food waste** without eating less

- 4 natural products you can use to make your own eco-friendly cleaning supplies

- The simple alternative to 'consumerism' — the age-old method for **getting what you need without paying money for it**

- The 9 fundamental items you need to create a self-sufficient first-aid kit

- One of the top skills that most people are afraid of learning — and how you can master it effortlessly

- 3 essential tips for **gaining financial independence**

The Prepper Emergency Preparedness & Survival Checklist:

10 Easy Things You Can Do Right Now to Ready Your Family & Home for Any Life-Threatening Catastrophe

Natural disasters demolish everything in their path, but your peace of mind and sense of safety don't have to be among them. Here's what you need to know...

- Why having an emergency plan in place is so crucial and how it will help to keep your family safe

- How to stockpile emergency supplies intelligently and why you shouldn't overdo it

- How to store and conserve water so that you know you'll have enough to last you through the crisis

- A powerful 3-step guide to ensuring financial preparedness, no matter what happens

- A step-by-step guide to maximizing your storage space, so you and your family can have exactly what you need ready and available at all times

- Why knowing the hazards of your home ahead of time could save a life and how to steer clear of these in case of an emergency

- Everything you need to know for creating a successful evacuation plan, should the worst happen and you need to flee safely

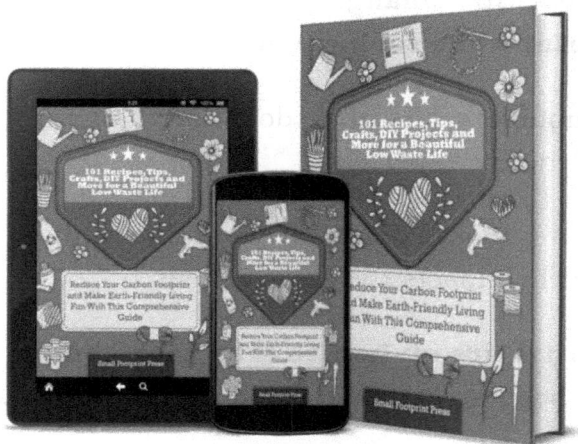

101 Recipes, Tips, Crafts, DIY Projects and More for a Beautiful Low Waste Life

Reduce Your Carbon Footprint and Make Earth-Friendly Living Fun With This Comprehensive Guide

Practical, easy ways to improve your personal health and habits while contributing to a brighter future for yourself and the planet

Discover:

- **Simple customizable recipes for creating your own food, home garden, and skincare products**

- The tools you need for each project to successfully achieve sustainable living

- Step-by-step instructions for life-enhancing skills from preserving food to raising your own animals and forging for wild berries

- **Realistic life changes that reduce your carbon-footprint while saving you money**

- Sustainable crafts that don't require any previous knowledge or expertise

- Self-care that extends beyond the individual and positively impacts the environment

- **Essential tips on how to take back control of your life -- become self-sustained and independent**

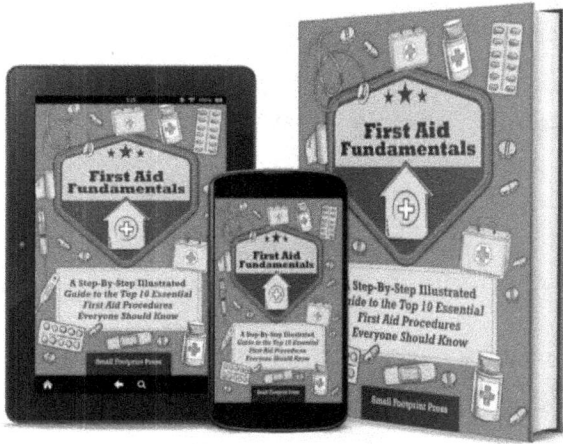

First Aid Fundamentals

A Step-By-Step Illustrated Guide to the Top 10 Essential First Aid Procedures Everyone Should Know

Discover:

- **What you should do to keep this type of animal attack from turning into a fatal allergic reaction**

- Why sprains are more than just minor injuries, and how you can keep them from getting worse

- **How to make the best use of your environment in critical situations**

- The difference between second- and third-degree burns, and what you should do when either one happens

- Why treating a burn with ice can actually cause more damage to your skin

- When to use heat to treat an injury, and when you should use something cold

- **How to determine the severity of frostbite**, and what you should do in specific cases

- Why knowing this popular disco song could help you save a life

- The key first aid skill that everyone should know — **make sure you learn THIS technique the right way**

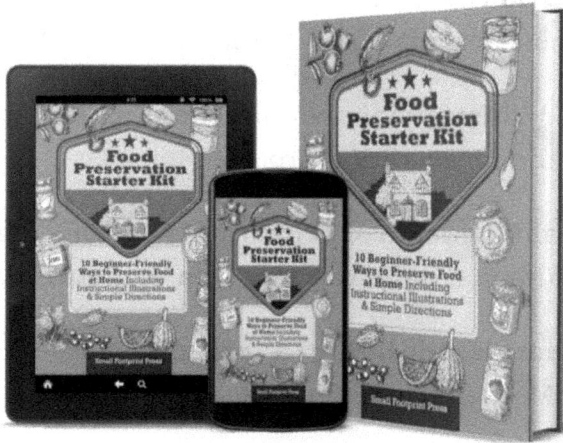

Food Preservation Starter Kit

10 Beginner-Friendly Ways to Preserve Food at Home | Including Instructional Illustrations and Simple Directions

Grocery store prices are skyrocketing! It's time for a self-sustaining lifestyle.

Discover:

- **10 incredibly effective and easy ways to preserve your food for a self-sustaining lifestyle**

- The art of canning and the many different ways you can preserve food efficiently without any prior experience

- A glorious trip down memory lane to learn the historical methods of preservation passed down from one generation to the next

- **How to make your own pickled goods**: enjoy the tanginess straight from your kitchen

- Detailed illustrations and directions so you won't feel lost in the preservation process

- The health benefits of dehydrating your food and how fermentation can be **the key to a self-sufficient life**

- **The secrets to living a processed-free life** and saving Mother Earth all at the same time

Download all your resources by scanning the QR-Code below:

SCAN ME

https://dl.bookfunnel.com/h8hzy33mn7

CONTENTS

THE GREAT SURVIVAL BOOK OF FORAGING WILD EDIBLE PLANTS

INTRODUCTION

"As dreams are the healing songs from the wilderness of our unconscious - So wild animals, wild plants, wild landscapes are the healing dreams from the deep singing mind of the earth."

– Dale Pendell

The adage, "Knowledge without practice is useless; practice without knowledge is dangerous," should be the motto for anyone entering the world of foraging wild plants for the first time. While the rewards of harvesting your own wild culinary and medicinal plants are enormous, there are very clear risks if you misidentify, mishandle, or misuse wild herbs. This is most true if a person relies on sources of information that are unverified.

One nature novice, eager to learn about herbs and experience using them first hand, read a blog post that indicated that thistle root was edible. The author talked about how he peeled and fried the thistle roots and how it tasted much like parsnip. Believing the information was reliable, the would-be harvester dug up a few thistles growing along the nearby roadside.

He cleaned and scrubbed the first few roots, but found them too small to peel. Then, he fried them in a little butter, as the blog writer had suggested. They were inedible—so tough that he couldn't chew them at all.

"Perhaps," he thought, "I should boil them first."

He boiled several roots, attempting to pierce them with a fork throughout the process. After forty minutes, the roots were no softer. He removed them and fried them again, just like the first batch. Every root had the consistency of tree bark. The taste was nothing like parsnips. They tasted like buttered cardboard.

There were myriad problems with this blind approach to eating wild-harvested plants. First, the article did not state which type of thistle to harvest. There were four species growing in the area. Second, he harvested the thistles in mid-summer, long after tender new plants had toughened. Third, the author of the post had no credible background in wild harvesting.

In North America, there are over 5,000 edible plants, according to various sources. But here, again, the internet is rife with conflicting data, some sites suggesting 25-50,000 edible species, others as few as 4,000. Worldwide, estimates suggest that there are 350,000 plant species, with anywhere between 20,000 and 80,000 being edible.

But what is edible? Some lichens may be edible, but hardly palatable. Some plants are not edible but have medicinal properties, such as members of the Saliaceae family (willow and poplar), whose inner bark contains a natural painkiller.

There are several dozen commonly consumed and used herbs in the western world, easily identified, harvested, and prepared. Some are so common that you may tread on them every day. A few are less common. A small number are on the endangered or near-endangered species list. Some have harmless look-alikes, others deadly cousins.

Here is where "practice without knowledge" is dangerous. But here, too, is where "wild plants ...are the healing dreams from the deep singing mind of the earth." With knowledge about identifying, harvesting, and preparing the herbs that you gathered in the wilderness, the experience becomes deeply gratifying and beneficial to your health, your pocketbook, and your general wellbeing.

Fortunately, learning about wild harvesting is a hands-on experience. You may start with just a few of the most common plants and, as you become comfortable with the experience, expand your arsenal of wild, healthy eating resources.

Did you know that wild fresh food can have over five times the nutrients that food in the store usually has? The further you venture into the wilderness to harvest, the more pristine your harvested foods will be, with fewer chemicals invading the habitat. Wild herbs "know" the best places to grow for their particular species, and produce more of the nutrients and essential oils, without artificial fertilizers, than similar plants in controlled commercial operations.

If you are a new wildcrafter, you may be nervous about venturing into this unfamiliar environment, worried that you might pick the wrong plant, unsure if you have the right herb or a poisonous look-alike. You may be concerned that the plants that you are harvesting are on an endangered list. Perhaps you worry if the plant actually provides the benefits that it is supposed to.

You may doubt that you will find the plants in the jumble of forest or meadow. Pickers that have never picked morel mushrooms may look for hours before they find the first morel and then, magically, dozens more may appear as soon as they identify the first one. If you are an inexperienced outdoors person, it may be easy to wander off a known route and get lost as you immerse yourself in picking.

These doubts and fears are normal for newcomers to harvesting food in the wild. This book will guide you, step-by-step, through identifying the habitat and range of various edible plants, look-alikes, and when to harvest.

The benefits of foraging extend beyond the nutritional, culinary, or medicinal benefits of the herbs you collect. Science has proven that nature is an excellent medicine for depression, stress, and lethargy. Spend time regularly outdoors and you will feel more energized and invigorated by fresh, unpolluted air.

Your wallet is healthier, as you save money that you would otherwise spend on forced-grown produce, often laden with chemicals, heavy metals, and toxins.

As you harvest your own wild food, you will find each step becomes easier until it is an absolute joy to know, finally, what you eat, where to find the best and freshest herbs every day, how to prepare the most nutritious meals from wild plants, and how to take control of your food budget without depending on lower-quality goods available from commercial growers.

Subsequent chapters reveal how and where to forage, safety measures to follow when identifying, picking, and handling your new foods, good conservation practices, and meals and medicinal remedies you can prepare with your fresh food basket.

Our guide provides you with easy-to-follow steps on your journey. The acronym, **F.R.E.S.H.S.** should help you remember each one, chapter by chapter.

F: **F**oraging, why forage, tools for foraging, and foraging guidelines.

R: **R**isk-free safety guidelines when foraging and handling wild herbs.

ESH: **E**dible **S**pecies of wild **H**erbs, available virtually in your backyard.

S: **S**ustainably harvesting and **S**toring your herbs.

There is no food like FRESH food, and no better way to improve your diet and your health than foraging!

ABOUT THE AUTHOR

Who is Small Footprint Press?

Small Footprint Press, established amidst the pandemic, is a self-publishing company of experts that aims to promote sustainable survival–equipping you to live a sustainable, conscious, and independent lifestyle to make the world a better place for yourself and future generations to come.

As the world progresses, we believe that the importance of sustainable survival becomes more and more evident. Our planet faces various challenges, including climate change, dwindling resources, population growth, and pandemics. To secure a bright future for our children, *now* is the time we must take steps toward saving our planet.

We accomplish this by simply empowering you to prepare for potential disasters for yourself and your loved ones. Gone are the days when you stress about the day of the unknown!

Our books are a collaboration of different authors, each with their perspective and expertise. This makes for a well-rounded book that covers various topics in-depth, ensuring the highest quality standards. It also makes for a more engaging read, as each author brings their style to the table.

Similarly, orchestras are made up of different instruments, each with its unique sound and purpose. Once these instruments play as one in harmony, the result is extraordinary.

We believe that one way to bridge a community of people with a shared purpose and values is through books! In this community, you build genuine relationships, share similar experiences, and are empowered to take action.

You are not alone. There's something special about a journey taken with others. Whether exploring a new city or embarking on a long hike, sharing the experience with others makes you enjoy the journey more than the destination.

So allow us to join you in your journey to a compelling life of sustainable survival!

Interested in joining our cause? Download your FREE resources at the beginning of the book!

CHAPTER ONE:
FORAGING 101

A fable written by Lucy Sprague Mitchell in 1948 told the tale of a little engine that was eager to get out on the tracks and begin traveling, but its mother kept telling him, "Steady, steady, 'til you're ready. Learn to know before you go." It was the essence of being prepared. It is possibly the most appropriate lesson as you prepare to forage in the wild for plants. Learn to know, before you go out into the woods.

There are lots of reasons why you should research, read about, and practice foraging for wild herbs with an experienced wildcrafter before you even consider striking out on your own. But you should also be asking yourself, "Am I ready?" "What do I still need to know?" "Why is it that I want to forage?"

Before you began your working life, you went through a number of tests and lessons in school that helped prepare you for the outside world of business. Now, you are contemplating a venture into the true outside world of nature. It has been waiting for you, and others, forever, but most of us have turned away from the bounty that it offers and have lost the knowledge that we need to enjoy its cornucopia. Prior to heading out, you need to make sure you are ready.

EXERCISE ONE: ARE YOU READY FOR FORAGING?

Take the time to answer the following questions to see how prepared you may be, and how much work you may still need to do, to become ready, capable, and even proficient at harvesting wild plants. We have offered a few guidelines to accompany each question, so you may further assess your readiness.

A. PERSONAL PHYSICAL READINESS

Foraging can test your stamina. It is more than just the trek into the wilds. Bending to pick or dig, wending your way through the underbrush, slogging through sloughs, and battling insects, all can test your physical and mental endurance. Many indigenous people of North America still dig Seneca root, which they sell to pharmaceutical manufacturers. It involves up to fourteen hours per day, bending, digging, and breaking clumps of mud. They toil in the hot sun, battle rain, and fight off mosquito hordes. They suffer.

Ask yourself, how much effort am I willing to expend? Then plan your day in the fields accordingly. Limit your hours of picking and the conditions under which you toil.

Questions: How good is your health? What sort of limits will you impose on all of your foraging excursions?

B. MOTIVATION

The idea of picking your own foods has a romantic appeal. It also likely has a practical appeal. Wild foods have a long history of use, medicinally and nutritionally. However, the convenience and the ability to get clean, unblemished, nicely packaged commercial foods at your nearby grocery also has appeal, since it is easier, faster, and the grocer's products are very familiar.

Perhaps you want to save money on medicinal herbs to replace expensive pharmaceuticals and culinary plants to supplant bought produce. Maybe you want to try some heritage recipes, using the ingredients that the pioneers used in the wild. Do you want to break away from relying on store-bought goods? Maybe you are just looking for a hobby and love the idea of spending more time outdoors.

Questions: What are your reasons for foraging? Are you looking for healthier options? Are you looking for creative cooking ideas or alternative medicines? Is this a hobby, combining exercise and healthy eating?

C. FINANCIAL & TIME CONSTRAINTS

Foraging is cheap. No huge growing conglomerate controls what you pick, and no retailer sets a price on the free food you gather. Foraging is healthy, with wild foods having few or none of the chemicals introduced to commercially grown crops and far more of the natural nutrients. Foraging is an experience, as you seek out, identify, verify, and pick your desired plants, instead of selecting the prettiest package of veggies in the produce aisle. Although, foraging is time-consuming. A fifteen-minute trip to the corner store may become a day-long trek into the wilderness.

Questions: Are you looking for ways to become more self-sufficient? Are you looking to eat with less expense? Are you looking to replace health supplements with free natural remedies? Do you have the time to set aside weekly, daily, or monthly to forage (and how much time)?

D. ACCESS TO THE WILDERNESS

A well-worn adage claims that golf is a 'good walk, spoiled.' Foraging is actually a great way to break up a good wilderness hike and embrace nature. Some of us are ill-suited to being in nature. We may have allergies, be uncertain about insects and predators, be reluctant to venture into unknown or unfamiliar areas. If so, we may want to rethink the idea of foraging. If, however, you like the outdoors, love hiking, enjoy exercise, understand and embrace nature, foraging is likely for you.

Many urban dwellers do not have access to rural spaces where foraging is safe and productive. Many areas may have an abundance of the plants you want, but they are growing in unsafe or polluted ground. Some areas may have the herbs you want, but they are in limited supply in those places. Many spots may be difficult to access. Ask yourself the following questions to see, not if you are ready for the wilderness, but if the wilderness and you are ready for each other.

Questions: Do you like hiking and have the necessary gear for it? Do you have an area already in mind for your excursion? Do you have the resources to be able to identify where to find your plants and know you have the right to access them?

E. Your Cohorts

Never pick alone. It is like swimming by yourself; it may not be safe, regardless of how experienced you may be. You may be quite capable of surviving on your own, but injuries can occur, particularly in regions where there are venomous or predatory animals. Even the most experienced trekkers can get lost. Maybe the risk is low, but hiking and picking with a cohort—friend or family—is advisable. It also is a great opportunity for bonding and is a wonderful way for your children to learn about wild harvests.

Questions: Can you involve your family in foraging? Do you have friends who will spend the time foraging with you? Does their schedule fit your timetable?

We introduced you to the concept of F.R.E.S.H.S. in foraging earlier. This chapter examines the practice of **F**oraging, or wildcrafting. We will explore the nutritional difference between foraged and cultivated plants, the reasons why you should forage, the where and how to forage, mindful foraging guidelines, and essential foraging tools.

WHAT IS WILD FOOD?

Wild food traditionally has included fish, game, some minerals, and plants. However, for the vegetarian and most pickers, wild food is completely herbal—edible plants.

The term "plants" is used in the botanical sense, referring to any of the flora in the region. It includes berries, fruits, vegetables, and leafy plants. The emphasis in this book is on edible plants. Worldwide, the number of edible plants may exceed 50,000, but usually is calculated at ten percent of the more than 350,000 plants in total. That also includes more than 2,000 edible mushrooms alone!

There is some confusion in the world of the wild harvester as to what the difference between "herbs" and "plants" may be. Some purists insist that an herb is any plant that does not have a stem and that dies down to the ground each season. Yet, that would exclude most tropical herbs, shrubs that produce berries or have usable bark (poplar and willow) or sap, cinnamon, teas, and a myriad other plants that are grouped into culinary or medicinal herb categories.

In this book, we may refer to some species as herbs, simply because that is what they are known as by many people, but we will largely adhere to referring to the thirty-two flora on which we focus as "edible plants."

NUTRITIONAL DIFFERENCES BETWEEN WILD AND CULTIVATED PLANTS

Wild foods are packed with more nutrients than their cultivated counterparts. In the wild, plants grow in conditions according to their needs. This difference in garden plants is partly the result of cultivation, focusing on taste over quality when domestic plants are bred and developed, with the desire to have a plant that produces quickly and with a greater output of edible parts. Gardeners and botanists often hybridize cultivated plants and modify them to increase production and speed up the growing process. These genetic adaptations result in a plant that does not have to be as hardy as a wild plant, losing many of the defense mechanisms that are inherent in the nutrient density of the wild counterpart.

For example, wild bitter herbs are much more powerful than cultivated versions, since they must deal with predators (insects and animals) that would eradicate them if not for a strong and bitter taste to deter pests. Plants growing in marginal soils need to store essential oils to survive seasons of deprivation and cold winters, while domestic versions are protected and often more tender.

This need to "be tougher" extends throughout the wild kingdom, from plants to insects to large animals. And tough means more of the nutrients and beneficial elements packed into a leaner survivor of the wild.

Because of the more intense qualities of wild crops, they also possess the adaptability needed to survive. They may have poisonous look-alikes, or bristles, thorns, irritants, and spears to hurt you. They may grow among other plants, like the poison trinity of oak, ivy, and sumac, or wind closely with other plants and roots to make them difficult to pick or dislodge, like wild ginger.

Hardy plants also tend to be scarcer and at risk of becoming endangered, as civilization, pollution, and climate change encroach. Be careful, not just for your own safety, but for the safety and survival of the plants themselves. Pick only what you need, for the shortest possible duration. A good guide is to pick no more than one-fifth of the available plants if abundant and one-tenth if they are more scarce.

Because you are foraging in areas that are new to you and for plants that you likely have not consumed recently, you are adding diversity to your diet. However, simply by wildcrafting, you are capitalizing on the greater diversity of nutrients and phytochemicals that wild plants contain. Nutritional diversity is very important for your overall health. This is because different foods have different macro-and micronutrients that the body's tissues need.

Cultivated plants exist in soils that are amended with fertilizers and synthetic chemicals, while wild plants draw on the natural soil and water reserves that have not been altered intentionally. This foundation contains more of the minerals needed for the growth of that specific plant. However, as air pollution increases, even the atmosphere contains chemicals that infiltrate into the wild, while runoff and rain often leaches heavy metals and chemicals from polluting industries and pushes them into the waterways.

Knowing where you are harvesting, therefore, is important, to avoid those harmful pollutants and to maximize the likelihood of picking pure, healthy, and nutrition-packed plants.

All reputable food guides recommend diet diversity. In the same way that a healthy immune system requires antibodies that combat a diverse range of viruses, bacteria, and illnesses, a diverse diet helps to create an adaptable, flexible, and strong body and mind. One of the reasons for the success of recognized diets like the Mediterranean diet is its emphasis on diversity, as well as nutrient-packed foods.

Of all the components of a healthy diet, as specified by the Mediterranean diet and the DASH (Dietary Approaches to Stop Hypertension) diet, and by the various food guides issued by countries around the world, plant-based foods top the lists.

The Nordic Council of Ministers claims that "observed health effects associated with vegetable, fruit, berry, and whole grain consumption can likely be explained by the combined action of many different phytochemicals and other nutrients" (Nordic Nutrition Recommendations 2012. Copenhagen: Nordic Council of Ministers).

Healthy diets today are more than the meat, starch, and vegetable basics of the 1950s. Protein, fatty acids, vitamins, and minerals form the basis of our needs, but our ever-expanding knowledge of the requirements that our bodies and minds have for healthy maintenance and growth continues to reveal new essential elements that interact with others to keep us alive.

WHY FORAGE?

Foraging is the super exercise of nature lovers. It provides immense benefits for your physical health, your dietary needs, mental health, intellectual growth, emotional wellbeing, and desire to explore new areas and gain new experiences—and it is very economical!

Foraging requires energy and physical endurance. There is a lot of bending, carrying, climbing, trekking, and exploring involved in this daytime adventure. Without realizing it, you may get the entire recommended quota of calisthenics or the steps that your Fitbit or fitness app urges you to get while you are out and about hunting. It is good for the heart, the lungs, the muscles, the joints, and the brain.

Of course, the gathering of food means you are taking care of your dietary needs, but on top of that, most mental health experts acknowledge and encourage the experience of visiting nature as a superb natural stress reliever. It has been shown, countless times, to help recharge your energy, both physical and mental. Unfortunately, many people today prefer to lock themselves indoors, and miss the healthy experience of being in nature.

As you forage, you learn. Yes, reading books can tell you what to expect, what to look for, but actual experience has always been the best teacher. You may be intent on learning about the plants that you are harvesting but, quite incidentally, you also will harvest a wealth of information about the rest of nature, its interactions, its survival mechanisms, and your role in protecting this wonderful world. It is mind-expanding. More so, even, than watching the best documentary about the wilderness because it is your personal experience that sustains this new knowledge.

More rewarding than being on a tropical holiday, an excursion into nature to forage brings great emotional satisfaction. It is your alone time with the world around you with no commercial intrusions. Your senses, as you trek, are heightened while you become more aware of all the activity and beauty you come into contact with.

As you explore, you will embrace the irresistible experience of needing to know more while more of the natural world surrounds you. Gaining new experiences may become as much a focal point as the foraging itself. All of this occurs in your own figurative backyard, with almost no cost. You may find yourself lost and immersed in this world, living only in the present moment.

WHERE TO FORAGE

Think of foraging as a scavenger hunt in the wilderness. You have specific plants in mind, but it is the joy of searching for them that provides the drive for your foraging practice.

One caution to consider: do not forage in urban areas! Pollutants that can invade your plants are everywhere, from the bug spray to pesticides used in nearby areas, from airborne industrial pollutants and vehicle exhausts to waterborne toxins and heavy metals in streams, ditches, and even in local acid rain.

You want to find pristine environments as much as possible. Unfortunately, some of your most powerful plants grow in wastelands, whether it is natural or manmade. Rural and woodside paths and hiking trails are generally much safer than urban locales, but they carry toxins that are borne on the footwear of hikers using the trails.

Even if you wash plants harvested in polluted environments, you will only cleanse away the surface toxins, not the chemicals and heavy metals that have become systemic in the plant.

The best places to forage are those that are most untouched and natural, such as woodlands and forests, meadows, and fields left fallow or uncultivated.

Many landowners and farmers would love to know that their property offers a bounty for wildcrafters like yourself, but it is vital that you get their permission. At the same time, inquire about their fertilizing and pest management habits so you know how safe your visit will be.

Golf courses and managed recreation areas often allow foraging and hiking, but be aware that golf courses have some of the highest uses of chemicals on their fairways, greens, and hazards. These likely get windblown into adjacent meadows and woods.

Public parks mostly do not prohibit picking, but be aware of their regulations. Always get permission, regardless of where you harvest. Check with park management, both upon arrival and departure. Developing a good relationship with the owners of favorite harvesting locations means you will be more welcome on your next visit.

Some foragers pay for the right to harvest in a particular location. This may cost a little more, but it guarantees that you know the quality of your crops and are able to maintain a reliable source, year after year.

One of the most productive sites to forage along is a waterway. These routes offer great diversity, as they may traverse forest and meadow, run through numerous states, be in sunlight or shade, and have their own varied ecosystems along their length. Soil variety and moisture diversity make for a wide array of different edible plants in ideal growing conditions.

There is one major problem for foragers who travel across the United States. From state to state, rules about riparian versus agrarian water rights differ, which makes knowing whether you have the ability to traverse these water routes difficult. Does the landowner own the water rights or is it in the public domain? Are you trespassing?

Plots of old western movies often revolved around a selfish or vengeful upstream owner shutting off the access to a vital stream for the farmer below. Most of the West has agrarian land rights, meaning that "shutting off the tap" is legal, as is denying access to people who want to use the stream to canoe.

In the eastern parts of the United States and Canada, riparian rights mean that the public can access the river and a certain right-of-way on its shore. In that instance, it is the state, province, or federal government that restricts or allows access and the privilege of harvesting along the shores of the waterway.

MINDFUL FORAGING GUIDELINES

Mindful foraging is self-explanatory, but takes time to become part of your conscious process. Be aware of how you forage, what you forage, where and when you forage, and what your responsibilities may be.

When you visit nature, you are experiencing an act of mindfulness and connection. But what the Earth gives to you, you should give back in some manner. Be sure to compost and recycle, be sure to use environmentally friendly practices, not just on your harvesting trip but in general.

The Earth's resources are limited. A once plentiful fish, Cod, is now only slowly recovering from its devastating over-harvesting history. Many prairie grasses and flowers are now extinct or almost so, as cultivated crops surge into their territory. The rainforests of the Amazon are also under extreme stress.

The saying, "leave no trace," is the perfect way to view your duties owed to nature as you enjoy her bounty.

Every summer, elders would join younger members of First Nations communities as they harvested, first Seneca root, then later in summer, wild rice. They joined the youth not because they loved the back-breaking work involved in these two harvests, but to teach the younger people their duty to the land.

Each plant has a season. During the flowering season, harvesting those plants would diminish the ability of that species to reproduce.

Elders would show students how to dig only the largest Seneca roots, leaving the younger plants to flower and produce seeds. In the fall, the crew might return to dig those roots that had the highest concentration of essential oils that the pharmaceutical company buyers wanted. But in all cases, they made sure that young proteges only took a tenth of the plants throughout the two digging seasons, so that the roots had several years to mature and several generations of seed to germinate.

Likewise, they only harvested a portion of the wild rice growing in the swamps and waterways, beating the grains into their canoes part-way through the period of ripening. In this way, immature seeds would continue to ripen after the team had departed, falling into the mud to reproduce. The indigenous tribes took only what they could use.

This mindfulness is at the core of most First Nations' spiritual beliefs. They are stewards of and have responsibility for the natural world around them.

There are plants that may be edible but are now endangered or near endangered. Across the Midwest, certain types of lady slippers are protected, yet they look very similar to other, unprotected varieties. If you are uncertain of the plant's status, don't harvest it. Ladyslipper's medicinal properties are tricky to make use of safely, and should be left alone regardless.

Leave no trace: no garbage, no damaged areas, no record of you being there. Correctly identify plants so that you do not later discover your error and discard them, when they could have been left to flourish.

Create a symbiotic relationship with nature and be grateful for its bounty.

Foraging Tools

The following is a list of tools that you will need when foraging:

1) *Pruners*: These shears are useful for woody stems and thicker stalks. Purchase good quality pruners with stay-sharp edges and grips that fit your hand comfortably, both when they are open and when they are closed.

2) *Hunting knife*: Some foragers swear they need a specific large blade knife. However, a durable hunting knife with a serrated edge for sawing is adequate. Make sure you have a good, safe sheath in which to contain it.

3) *Small digging fork (army style)*: Used to dig out intertwined roots (optional).

4) *Small, cut-off shovel (army style, not emergency camping quality)*: Needed only if you are harvesting roots.

5) *Kitchen scissors*: Vital for clipping leaves and stems without causing any damage to the rest of the plant.

6) *Vegetable brush*: For cleaning dirt and debris from harvested plant parts (optional).

7) *First aid and survival kit*: Always carry a basic first aid kit when in the wild, regardless of whether or not you are foraging.

8) *Cell phone with compass app*: Needed if you are in cell phone range, a compass and whistle are also helpful.

9) *Field guide*: Either a phone app or a paperback version to verify the identity of the plants that you are harvesting.

10) *Small hand magnifying glass*: To examine smaller leaves and markings you may find on plants (optional).

11) *Cloth bags*: To carry foraged items.

12) *Bug repellent*: Use environmentally friendly repellent. Ants and flying insects can be a problem, but we still want to 'leave no trace' in our foraging environments.

13) *Garden gloves*: Essential to prevent stings from insects, nettles, thorns, and nearby poisonous plants.

14) *Water*: Always have water with you, or at minimum, the chemical treatment for creek water, if you know there is a safe stream near where you are harvesting.

15) *A plan*: Tell others where you are going and when you will return.

CHAPTER TWO:

SAFETY FIRST

The American Association of Poison Control Centers reports that between 5,000 to 8,000 people are poisoned each year in the United States by mushrooms and plants, with eight to 18 deaths. But these statistics are at the low end of the scale as many incidents are not even reported or are misidentified. The majority of cases occur because the plants are misidentified or mistaken as being safe.

The movie *Into the Wild* chronicles the death of Chris McCandless, who died after eating wild potato seeds. He had no idea that the food was toxic. Thousands of people in France fall ill after eating poisonous mushrooms every year. Many of the toxic interactions with plants are not sufficiently serious to warrant medical intervention. Think of the hundreds of thousands of cases of poison ivy and poison oak across North America, or upset stomachs after drinking alcohol and eating certain mushrooms. Many plants cause contact dermatitis, yet also are edible or medicinally beneficial. Stinging nettle is a prime example.

In the past century, with all of the pollution of industry, the number of those suffering from respiratory issues such as Asthma has risen exponentially. These sensitivities compound already existing allergies, exaggerating peoples' sensitivity to plant pollens in the respiratory system and even heightening immune responses in general. More and more, allergies are arising to plant species that are generally helpful and healthy for the body.

Clearly, misidentifying and mishandling plants can cause health issues and allergic reactions. Yet some of those same plants may be vital to our health and wellbeing. For years Digitalis, a component of foxglove, was a vital heart medication, saving thousands of lives. Codeine, from poppy plants, exists alongside opium from the same herb. Phytochemicals from plants, many from the rainforests of South America and Africa, are the basis of dozens of commercial medications and the simple remedy Aspirin owes its entire existence to salicylic acid in willow bark.

Safety when foraging extends beyond the toxicity of plants. Consuming or even handling the wrong plant or a beneficial plant in the wrong way can have catastrophic consequences. There are concerns about physical safety in the wilderness, and coming to harm while you are foraging along roadsides or in fields. Man-made and introduced chemicals pose a huge risk if caution is not exercised.

Safety concerns are significant in the handling, picking, storage, and consumption of various plants. With each plant in the subsequent chapters, we will discuss specific handling and safety issues, as warranted.

At the start of the book, we talked about how important gathering knowledge is to the wildcrafter. In the same way that a wild animal mother teaches its young about risks in the environment, you should begin your journey as a forager of wild plants under the tutelage of someone with experience.

Many settlers in Canada and the United States would have perished if they had not benefited from the teachings and directions of First Nations in these areas. For example, the entire Icelandic settlement in Manitoba would not exist today, were it not for the guidance of a native man, John Ramsay, who risked his life to make sure that the newcomers knew how to live off the land during its harsh winters.

The Lakota Nation, seen in offensive roles in cough remedy ads, actually used the very natural remedies now being promoted for coughs and colds. Tribes from Washington state guided the explorers and surveyors, Lewis and Clark, showing them how to survive on what the land provided.

Joel, a neophyte forager, was astonished to learn that there were stinging nettle plants right in his own yard. His neighbor pointed to a couple of small immature plants along the fence, one less than eighteen inches high, the other a teenager at about two and a half feet. Eagerly, Joel reached down to grasp the taller plant, his gardening glove on his hand.

But he was wearing a tee shirt with short sleeves. As he grasped the base of the larger plant to look at it more closely, his bare arm came in contact with the smaller one. Immediately, he felt the sting and itch of the hairs on the small plant. He had read that young plants don't develop stings until they are more mature. Not knowing precisely when that was, he paid the price for disregarding safe foraging guidelines.

Relying on experience and knowledge is the best way to master your own ability to forage effectively and safely. In our acronym, F.R.E.S.H.S. we look next at the "**R**," or the concept of **R**isk-free, safe foraging. Safety is mostly common sense. We have laid out nineteen tips for you to follow to gather and consume wild herbs safely.

GENERAL GUIDELINES FOR FORAGING

There are key points to remember whenever you venture into the wild to forage:

1. **When you pick a plant, first be very sure that it is the right plant.** As you harvest, you may mix in each of your plants to be sorted, washed, prepared, and consumed once you return home. With some plants, just the smallest quantity of a toxic look-alike may cause severe health issues and it is extremely easy to accidentally mix a few loose leaves of a poisonous plant in with the harvest of other plants.

2. **Be aware of the soil and surrounding crop farming habits.** Pesticides and herbicides tend to travel with the wind, and headlands of crop fields are often laden with chemicals. If you are picking on walking trails in the bush, or along roadsides and abandoned homesteads, be sure you know if these areas have been subjected to chemical applications. Very often, rail lines and highway workers spray for insects or fast-growing weeds, rather than more sustainably handling the problem. Try to avoid picking anywhere chemicals might have been used. This is also true of creeks and streams, where pollutants may have entered the waterways further upstream.

3. **Make sure you have the landowner's permission to forage on the property where you pick.** Be very aware of boundaries. Some properties may be pastures for animals, some may be government-controlled preservation areas, and others may merely be property that the owner prefers to be free of any trespassers.

4. **Never take more than 25 percent of the visible supply of any plant**. Leave an abundance for nature to reproduce itself. This is particularly true with mushrooms or wild berries. With such a short season for picking, there is an urge to capitalize, but the more you pick, the less opportunity there is for reproduction. Remember, too, that you are sharing the wilderness with other animals and insects who need to feed as well.

5. **Be sure that you are not picking an endangered or at-risk species.** Many plants are being squeezed out of existence in some areas, and even though they may be abundant elsewhere, are threatened. Plants like wild bergamot, small white lady slipper, Hill's slipper, and Riddell's goldenrod, found in the tall grass prairies of Montana, the Dakotas, Saskatchewan, and Manitoba are at serious risk of extinction.

6. **Be aware of wild animal risks.** You are in their home. Be safe.

7. **Be weather-aware.** Sudden changes in temperature may catch you unawares, and in some parts of the continent flash flooding can occur in hours, or even less.

8. **Be aware of your location.** Know how to find your way in and out, and leave a detailed explanation at home as to where you are going and when you will be back.

9. **Carry reserves.** Be sure you have lots of water or access to clean drinking water. There are tablets that you can use to treat creek water, but you need containers in which to do so. Have enough food and survival equipment in case you get lost or delayed.

10. **Have a safety kit.** Accidents are unpredictable. If they were not, they would not be called accidents. Later, we provide a list of survival items to bring along with you.

11. **Carry a compass if you are not in cell phone range, and carry a solar charger for your phone if you are.** Install a compass app on your phone.

12. **Be aware of your surroundings at all times.** This is self-explanatory.

13. **Carry a field guide of local plants with you.** Recognize, too, that the range of many plants has extended dramatically in recent decades, with plants found in states and provinces where they never existed a century ago. If you are in cell phone range on your trek, consider downloading and using a plant identification app with photo recognition, such as Plant Snap. However, do not rely solely on this type of application, as it is possible to misidentify species and be less accurate.

14. **Avoid plants with a strong, disagreeable odor.** Many plants have an odor to warn predators away, skunk cabbage

being a prime example. Odor can be a warning for humans as well.

15. **Don't assume that if an animal eats it, it is safe for you.** Animals eat all kinds of things, would you? And many plants that we can eat, animals cannot. For instance, horsetail is poisonous to horses, but we can consume modest amounts. Most animals are not bothered by poison ivy, but most people are.

16. **"Leaves of three, let them be."** This well-known slogan for poison ivy and similar plants is self-explanatory, but many plants have similar leaf structures, and identifying which is which can take time. Be sure to focus on leaf structure, stem structure, and other subtle features of plants to really be able to identify.

17. **Raw Consumption**. Some plants, fungi and berries, like chokecherry and many mushrooms, should not be eaten raw.

18. **Potential Allergies.** Try small quantities of new plants first to make sure you are not allergic or intolerant. Like a test spot of paint, try a small test of a new food item to make sure you and your immune system find it to be agreeable.

19. **Poisonous neighbors**. When picking plants, be sure there are no poisonous ones nearby. Wear disposable or garden gloves when possible, because plant oils can spread and brush against you, even if you are not picking them

Follow these rules and you'll be safe! Read these tips over and over again until you commit them to memory.

There's no need to panic if you stick to these rules. Even when you think you know what you're doing, reconnect with humbleness and always question yourself to avoid picking the wrong herb or plant, or fruit. In this beginner-friendly book, the herbs provided are easy to recognize to get you started on your foraging journey!

GETTING STARTED WITH FORAGING

Do not rush into the world of foraging. Take time to read and learn. Join a local group and be part of their excursions before you venture out on your own. Take a course, whether in person or online. Watch nature documentaries. The more information that you have before you launch yourself into this new world of nutrition, the better your experience will be.

Remember, there really can be too much of a good thing! Never eat excessive amounts of anything, instead eat moderate amounts of wild plants or fungi. Small quantities may be safe, while large quantities may be toxic. Always be prepared. It is a famous motto, but applicable to many situations in life. In the world of foraging, it is vital to always be prepared, always be aware, always be cautious, and always keep safety at the top of your list of priorities.

CHAPTER THREE:

IDENTIFYING EDIBLE SPECIES OF WILD HERBS

How much do you know about wild herbs? What do you want to accomplish when you forage? Why do you want to harvest wild plants? Let's start with a short exercise for you to see where you are currently.

Questions:

1. Have you ever picked wild food?

2. Do you have prior knowledge of the quality and appearance of herbs?

3. Are you aware of their medicinal and culinary uses?

4. Do you have the time to learn about edible wild plants before you begin harvesting?

5. How much time, per week, do you normally spend outdoors and in nature?

6. Are you looking for a hobby that is healthy?

7. Do you want to become less reliant on commercial products?

8. Is your primary goal to eat healthier or discover medicinal uses for herbs?

9. Do you have access to, or can you identify locations where you can harvest safely?

10. Do you have a source or person who can assist you as you learn how to forage?

11. Do you have storage facilities for your edible plants?

Prior knowledge of the appearance of wild plants and an understanding of their value for cooking, nutrition, and medicinal qualities is beneficial. If you have picked and chewed on a dandelion leaf, sucked on a sorrel leaf when you were thirsty, or applied a plantain leaf to a cut or insect bite, you can appreciate the magical powers of wild herbs.

You might want to start small in your search for wild, natural foods. Plantain at the edge of your garden, nettle along the fence line of your property, purslane in your garden, or clover sprouting in your unfertilized lawn might be a good start.

Take the time to read books on wild plants, including the amazing mushroom family. Watch online or television documentaries on wild plants. Listen to opposing views about eating wild plants, so you will know that there are some risks associated with this new hobby.

While there is a wealth of anecdotal data regarding the benefits of eating wild foods, there are also those that claim that the benefits have not been scientifically proven. This may be true, but centuries of lore and practices provide a strong indication of the benefits of eating wild plants. Across continents, the practices of foraging and wild food are remarkably similar over hundreds of years of history. While we wait for science and the pharmaceutical industry to catch up with the knowledge of generations, we can assume that the plants are safe and likely to be beneficial as claimed.

If you don't spend much time outdoors, proceed slowly. Familiarize yourself with the concept of interacting with nature passively, then begin your active journey into gathering your food.

We are examining "E.S.H" in this chapter. You will be introduced to the anatomy of plants, and techniques to use that anatomy to identify "**E**dible **S**pecies of **H**erbs."

Consider your new food project both an opportunity to exercise and as a healthy hobby. It should not be looked upon as a task or tedious chore.

A desire for independence from commercial, contaminated, and chemically treated products has led millions of people to healthier eating, even if many are not foraging for their own food. Some may be turning to organic and free range growers, others to farmers markets to buy freshly picked wild herbs, or maybe picking their own to achieve greater independence.

Wild herbs are healthier than domestically grown ones and provide superior medicinal benefits. If this is your goal, it is one of the best reasons to harvest in the wild. But you need to identify the best areas to harvest, and you need to treat those sites with respect.

Work with a friend or someone with herbal knowledge at first. Then encourage family and friends to join you.

If you have been able to answer all of these questions positively, you are ready to begin your trek into the wild!

SEASONS AND TIMINGS OF PLANT HARVEST

Every herb has its season for harvesting, and each season varies with the region of the country in which you reside. Identifying those timelines will increase the likelihood of your success when foraging. Knowing when to go is as important as knowing where to go.

Plants whose leaves are the primary part harvested will often be ready within four to six weeks of sprouting in the spring, but some plants germinate or rouse from dormancy later than others. Seeds often are harvested in the late summer and fall, but some plants grow quicker than others. Root crops are harvested in the spring or late autumn, when the essential oils and nutrients are still concentrated in those parts of the plant. Fruit may be ready early to mid-summer.

We have included the prime harvest seasons for each plant we describe in subsequent chapters.

STEPS TO IDENTIFY PLANTS

Know plants' habitats. Each of the 32 chapters on herbs in this guide describes the regions in which they grow and the type of conditions in which they can be found.

Once you have located the habitat, range, and season of a plant, you will identify the physical characteristics of that plant: flower anatomy, leaf shape, stem, growing habits, and even root style.

Here is where a field guide book or identification app on your phone is invaluable. One such application is Plant Snap. Take a picture of the plant, and the app automatically identifies its most likely species and family. Neither book nor application are foolproof, but they could save you from misidentifying and possibly encountering a poisonous look-alike.

PLANT ANATOMY

Almost all plants have basic parts that, although varied in appearance, make up the entirety of the plant. Plants in the same family will have similar certain parts that will help you in their identification.

These parts are the root, stem, leaves, and flowers. As the plant matures, flowers may become fruits, some having seeds contained, while others simply produce seeds or spores.

Identification of plants involves knowing root type (tuber, rhizome, tap, etc.), stem type (square, round, ribbed, etc.), leaf shape (oval, tapered, serrated, etc.), flower description (cross, bell, funnel, etc.), and fruit or seed description (cone, tubular, spore, etc.).There are diverse ways that a plant may propagate, including rhizomes, runners, seeds, or spores.

The way a plant reproduces has been a classification marker for scientists organizing the botanical world. Whether a plant produces fruit, spreads by rhizome or more can be a very good way to identify to which group it belongs.

Any part of a plant in general, may be edible, but each plant has edible and non-edible parts, some toxic, some non-lethal but deterrent, and others simply unpalatable.

Many look-alikes may be harmless, while others may be irritating, toxic, or poisonous. Using the specific plant descriptions, you will need to be able to identify one from the other.

Roots

Primary root types in the plant world are tap, fibrous, and adventitious.

Taproots are easily identified. They are found in common vegetables like carrots, beets, turnips, and parsnips. Similar root-heavy wild plants would be wild carrot, or burdock.

Adventitious roots are a little peculiar, in that they usually arise from the stem and may be partially in the air before entering the ground. They include rhizome roots, tubers, and aerial-origin roots like corn.

The most common root is the fibrous root. The root arises from the base of the stem and has a multitude of branching root parts, mostly of equal diameter. These are the roots most often found in grasses and in many rainforest trees.

All three types have family members whose roots are edible.

There are other varieties of roots, including those of parasitic plants and aerial roots. Mushrooms and other fungi produce spores for reproduction but are interconnected by mycelia, which run underground through a fine network in mossy or decaying material soils.

STEMS

Many plant families have unique stems that aid in identifying them. Some of these shapes are so similar to others that it may be difficult to distinguish them. Others may have stunted or almost non-existent stems (like some fungi), others have stems that are so undeveloped that they do not appear to be stems, such as low-growing, creeping plants.

The primary shapes of plant stems are square, angular, oval, lens, triangular, round, winged, ribbed, fluted, hollow, spines, thorns, prickles, and hairs.

When examining an unfamiliar plant, it is advisable not to handle them until you are certain that they are not poisonous, toxic, or irritant. If possible, carry and use disposable nitrile gloves when handling new plants in the wild.

Square–This stem is easy to identify. All members of the mint family have square stems. By rolling the stem between your fingers, you can verify its shape easily. While others, such as fluted stems, may seem similar, the square feel of the mint family stem has no variation along its length.

Angular–These stalks or stems, when cut in a cross-section, have more than four sides and may be ridged or hollow. They include daisies, horehounds, and hops.

Oval–These appear in the cross section to be an elongated or flattened circle. They are more common in wet environments and include bladderwort and pondweed.

Lens–Lens-shaped stems look something like the lens of an eye, almost almond-shaped. Plants with lens-shaped stalks include many irises.

Triangular–Triangular stems have only three sides. Some plants with angular stalks are garlic, bilberry, arrowhead, and sedges.

Round–As the name suggests, round stems are uniformly round, but can be ridged, hollow, or furrowed. Many plants have round stems in varying thicknesses. Sunflower is one such plant, and several of the creeping plants, such as creeping Charlie, also have round stems.

Winged–This stem most often has a round core, and sometimes square, but the flutes actually protrude like wings. They may also spiral around the stem. They may have two or more 'wings'. Thistles and comfrey commonly have winged stems.

Ribbed–Ribbed stems can be any core shape but have ribs or ridges on them. Bearberry, artichoke, aster, clover, and horsetail have ribbed stems.

Fluted–Fluted stems are distinguishable in our garden, with many having concave shapes. These include celery, rhubarb, and wormwood.

Hollow–Hollow stems, as the name says, have hollow cores. Often, they contain a sap. They include milk thistle, spurge, nettle, and dandelion.

Spines–There are several subcategories of spiny stems. These include thorns, prickles, and hairs. Generally, spiny stems have protrusions that can scratch, prick, or irritate when in contact with skin. Thorny plants include hawthorn, blueberry, and rose. Prickly plants include prickly pear cactus, wild cucumber, and thistle. Hairy plants include nettle.

LEAVES

The easiest way to identify a plant is through its leaf structure and shape.

The parts of a leaf that will provide a guide to identification are the base, margins, lamina, veins, tip, petiole, and midrib. The most telling parts of the leaf are its shape and arrangement.

The leaf may be simple or compound, palmate, pinnate, or bi-pinnate, and any of a range of shapes from round to oblong, needle to tapered.

Leaf color may vary from gray to bright green, purples and pinks to hues of blues.

Lastly, leaf texture helps in identification. Smooth, waxy, hairy, limp, and thick are a few terms used to describe texture.

Bases

The base is the part of the leaf that attaches to the stem. It may be sheathed (wheat), or appear indistinguishable from the petiole. Most protect a small bud in the axil. Some flare at the bottom, like those in legumes such as clovers.

Petiole: the leaf stalk that pushes out the leaf lamina so that it can obtain sunlight. It only exists in some, not all plant leaves.

Lamina: the thin, generally flat, and widened part of the leaf. Many plants have a central vein in the leaf, called a midrib. From it, several branching veins may be evident, and number and pattern of veins can be an excellent point of identification for plant species.

Veins

The central vein of a leaf is known as the midrib, but it is part of the leaf vascular system similar in purpose to our lungs or veins and arteries.

Midrib arrangement may consist of a singular, central midrib vein or more than one equally dominant vein. They are known as pinnate or palmate (like a palm of the hand with fingers) with more than one dominant vein.

Pinnates have one dominant rib with minor veins running away from the central vein.

Palmates may be of two types: divergent or convergent. When the veins branch out away from the base and then converge again at the top, they are convergent (willow). When they diverge from the base and do not route back toward each other, they are divergent (maple).

Parallel Venations are more uncommon. Veins run parallel to each other, away from the central midrib. Plants with this vein structure include thatch palm and many ferns.

Arrangement and Composition

Leaves may be either simple or compound, and within those categories there are subgroups.

A *simple pinnate leaf* is when the incision of the lamina flows toward the midrib, like the leaf of a turnip.

A *simple palmate leaf* is when the incision of the lamina flows toward the petiole, such as the leaf of a castor plant.

A *compound leaf* is broken up into several segments, like separate small leaves on one stem. Ash, Rose, or Elder trees have compound leaves. There are two types of compound leaves: *pinnately compound* and *palmately compound*, which, in turn, have subcategories.

Pinnately compound leaves have a number of leaflets, either arranged alternately or in an opposite manner. Four sub-categories of pinnately compound leaves are unipennate, bipinnate, tripinnate, and decompound.

Unipennate leaves send out leaflets directly from the midrib, *bipinnate leaves* send out secondary axes with leaflets on them, *tripinnate leaves* send out another level of leaves from axes sprouting from the secondary ones, and *decompound leaves* have more than three levels, like carrots and coriander.

Palmately compound leaves have one or more leaflets attached to the peak of the lamina, with these leaflets in the primary stage of development.

Shape

Leaves may be arranged on the stem of a plant in many ways. They can be *opposite, alternate opposite, whorled,* and also in a *simple* configuration.

They may be *lobed* (like in the oak or maple leaf), *toothed & serrated* (like a cherry or holly leaf), or *entire* with shapes like round, oblong, tapered, and pointed.

Evergreen (coniferous) trees and shrubs (like rosemary, pine, spruce, fir, yew) may have *single needles* like the spruce and fir, or *cluster* and *bundle needles* like the pines.

Ovate leaves are egg-shaped and wider at the stalk, *obovate leaves* are tear-shaped, with the taper at the stalk, *lanceolate leaves* look like lance tips, *acute leaves* are long, slightly oval, and pointed at the tip, *rhomboids* are triangular-shaped, and *spatulate* are shaped like a spatula.

There are other "telling" descriptors of the leaf that often are referred to as parts of the leaf. They include margins and tips.

Margins–edges of the leaf may be smooth, jagged, or saw-toothed. Crenate leaves have rounded teeth along the edges, dentate leaves have sharp teeth-like shapes on the edges, serrated leaves look like the teeth of a saw blade, and undulates have wavy edges or margins.

Tips–this part of the leave may be round, pointed, or split.

FLOWER ANATOMY

A grade school mnemonic phrase says, "Stamen, Stigma up, I have a Pistil here, and it's just my Style. I asked a question, and I want an Anther." It may sound silly, but you will remember the basic reproductive parts of a flower now!

Stamen—the male organ of the flower

Stigma—the head of the pistil

Pistil—the female organ of the flower

Style—the stalk of the pistil

Anther—the head of the stamen.

Most plants can be identified by the flower, in addition to stalks, roots, and leaves.

The remaining parts of the flower, from the stem to the tip of the flower, are peduncle, receptacle, sepal, ovary, filament, and petal.

The peduncle is the extended part of the stalk of the flower, leading into the receptacle in which the flower sits, the sepal, or cage green parts of the receptacle that hold the rest of the flower, ovary (which holds the flower's "eggs"), filament (part on which the anther sits holding it to the flower) and petals. Petals, of course, are the identifiable "pretty" parts of the flower that will help attract pollinators.

It is the shape and arrangement of the petals and entire petiole that distinctly identify a specific flowering plant.

Flower Shapes

There are two broad types of flower shapes: round and symmetrical (or tubular). Within each type, there are several common shapes you will come across.

Saucer-shaped: large, broad petals close together, forming a shallow bowl shape. These mostly are insect-pollinated or wind-pollinated.

Cup-shaped: more concave version of the saucer shape. Many insects must crawl into these.

Cross-shaped: four petals make up the flower, arranged at ninety degrees to each other.

Star-shaped: five or more distinct petals radiating outward.

Slipper-shaped: a version of a tubular shape formed like a slipper. They are more delicate and generally abundant in nectar and pollen. They are relatively uncommon in temperate climates.

Bell-shaped: these have a deeper narrower bowl than cup-shaped but are often smaller. The petals tend to splay outward at their tips, forming a bell shape.

Tubular-shaped: these often have a pipe-like shape or tall champagne glass appearance.

Funnel-shaped: a loosely packed adaptation of the tubular shape with the petals fanning slightly outward.

Pitcher-shaped: these flowers have a bulbous, wide bottom of the flower tapering towards the top into a cone shape.

Trumpet-shaped: they have a funnel shape at the base, with the petals opening gently out from halfway to resemble a trumpet. They often droop downward.

Rosette-shaped: these flowers have several rows of tightly packed flowers formed in whorls or in circles.

Pompom: a more complex rosette shape taken to extremes with the rows curling back to form a ball. Examples are hydrangeas or German statice.

Pea-like: an unsymmetrical shape, with one large upper petal, two medium side ones, and two small petals at the bottom. Examples are the sweet pea.

Petal Arrangements

Wildflowers have the most basic petal arrangements. As plants were hybridized and bred for appearance, they became more complex and ornamental. There are six primary arrangements:

Single: this is the simplest petal layout, with a single row of fairly flat petals. They are often the flowers of wild plants.

Recurved petals: these petals curve backward from the central point, exposing the stamens prominently, like the tiger lily or wild columbine.

Reflexed petals: similar to recurved, but with straighter petals pointing backward. They are designed to attract flying insects for pollination.

Semi-double petals: less common in the wild, since they tend to be the result of plant breeding. They have two or three rows of petals, forming a typical rose shape.

Double petals: they have several rows of petals forming a tight, layered circle, with few visible stamens. These flowers generally produce abundant pollen and less nectar.

Fully double petals: hybrid petunias, cosmos, or other cultivated flowers fit this grouping. They have a dense dome or ball of petals, often with no visible stamens at all.

Flower Groupings

Flowers are grouped in several ways.

Solitary: each flower is a single flower on one stalk. These include tulips.

Cluster: several flowers, each with a single straight stalk originating on the same stem point. Orchids form cluster flowers.

Flowerhead: many smaller, stalkless florets bunched across a flattened disc. Daisies have a flowerhead.

Umbel: like a cluster, but the numerous flowers form a bowl shape from a single point on the tip of the stem. Carnations form an umbel.

Spike: multiple stalkless flowers growing very densely outward from a single stem. These include larkspur and purple loosestrife.

Raceme: one single primary stem, producing multiple side stalks each with one flower. Gladiolas are racemes.

Cyme: each stem contains several side stalks with several flowers each, like a bluebell.

Corymb: a dense cluster of single-flowered stalks emerging from different parts of the primary stem. They form a dome or flat-topped cluster resembling a single flower. Mints have lovely corymb flowers.

Panicle: the most complex arrangement of flowers, with combinations of raceme, cyme, or corymb clusters branching from the primary stem. Many rangy, thin, prairie flowers have this panicle arrangement.

Flower Habits

Flower habits are the ways the flowers hang from their stalks. Habits may change as the flower grows. The following descriptions are for mature habits.

Erect: all the flower parts point straight upward. These are some of the most common and include daisies and crocuses.

Horizontal: the entire flower points to the side at right angles to the stem, such as gladiolus and some sedge-grasses.

Nodding: as the name suggests, these flowers point loosely downward from an upright stem. The weight of the flowers bends the stem down. Clematis and nodding onion are two types of nodding flowers.

Pendent: typical of bluebells, the entire flower hangs vertically downward from a horizontally pointing stem.

Flower Color Types

There are four general groups of color types and patterns.

Self-colored: this is the most common variety of flower colors. The color is uniform and singular across the entire flower. Scarlet lightning is self-colored.

Bicolored: these flowers have two distinct colors in each petal, with a clear division between base and tip. These are features bred into the flower, and so are found in highly hybridized or cultivated plants. It can happen spontaneously in many species. Some zinnias are bicolored.

Picotee: these are a variant of bicolored flowers with the edge showing a different color than the rest of the petals.

Striped: striped flowers containing two colors in stripes along the length of the petal include the cascade petunia and some complex domestic roses.

With all these subtle parts of the plant, the best way to dig into identifying and finding wild plants is to examine each species. Below you will find a list of thirty-two recognizable and foragable plants from across North America. This collection is by no means exhaustive, but you will find a wide variety of uses and some which you already recognize from your own backyard.

CHAPTER FOUR:

ASPARAGUS

Latin Name: Asparagus officinalis

It is easy to understand asparagus' symbolic connection to fertility from early Roman times, onward. The phallic symbol originally grew in the gardens of rich citizens of Rome. In addition to its reputation as an aphrodisiac, it is a symbol of birth and rejuvenation, being one of the first green shoots of every spring. When introduced to England, folklore claimed that it was known simply as "a spear of grass," eventually shortened to a-spear-a-grass, or asparagus.

Ironically, it is also a symbol of order and status, given its short harvest season, quick growth, and the history of being only available to aristocrats, but it has become somewhat of a barbarian plant, growing wild in every region of the United States.

Dioscorides, a very early author of books on plants, claimed that if one planted bits of ram's horns, asparagus would spring up. Of course, it even seemed unlikely to him! He further claimed that wearing an amulet of upside-down asparagus would make one barren, while Arabic health experts 1200 years later claimed that the same method would increase carnal lust and improve a person's fertility.

This historical and amusing discordance ties well into the "love-it-or-hate-it" attitude adopted in the modern-day about asparagus.

Description of the Plant: asparagus is readily identified by its spear-like stems and leaves rolled as if one. The spears grow from the base of the plant in early spring. In early summer, flowers emerge along the length of these stems. At this point, they are woody and inedible.

Common Names: it is known as sparrow grass and asparagus fern.

How, When, and Where to Gather: wild asparagus can be found in every state of the United States and every province of Canada, growing as far north as the 54th parallel. It is not native to North America, it was introduced in Europe as a cultivated crop and brought to the Americas with colonization.

It grows best in black soils, grassy meadows, vacant lots, gravelly areas along pathways and roadways, waste areas, and fence rows. It prefers sandy soils that have been disturbed.

Asparagus is best picked in early morning and in spring, when moisture content is high and plants remain tender.

Health, Nutritional, and Medicinal Benefits: it is an antioxidant, anti-inflammatory, antibacterial, antihepatotoxic, immunostimulant, anticancer, diuretic, and laxative.

Asparagus, aside from being a very healthy culinary vegetable, has health benefits that include being a laxative, having contraceptive effects, acting as a treatment for neuritis, cancer, rheumatism, acne, UTIs, kidney and bladder stones, constipation, anemia, and AIDs.

Edible Parts: the stem/leaves or the singular shoot that appears above the ground can be eaten and enjoyed.

Look-Alike Plants (Poisonous and Not): asparagus' fruits are poisonous–Japanese knotweed, horsetail, asparagus fern, and blue indigo all look like asparagus. Only blue indigo is poisonous.

Recipe: **Wild Asparagus Salad**

Ingredients

½ pound wild asparagus, washed, trimmed

2 eggs, hard-boiled and crumbled

⅓ teaspoon paprika

2 tablespoons parmesan cheese

Salt & pepper to taste

Method:

Boil asparagus for three to five minutes until slightly tender. Cool, add spices, top with egg, and cheese.

CHAPTER FIVE:

BLACKBERRY

Latin Name: Rubus allegheniensis

Blackberries carry a heavy burden of folklore and spirituality that does not rest well with this highly nutritious and tasty berry.

Legend says that Lucifer was thrown out of heaven on September 29–Michaelmas Day–and he landed in a big patch of brambles. He cursed the brambles from that day on, spitting on them, scorching them, and swore that those that ate blackberries after that date would be cursed. So, if legends are to be believed, buy or pick blackberries in October with extreme caution! Why then are we allowed to eat the fruit the rest of the year, if Satan spit, urinated, and stomped on them?

And why, in some parts of the world and Christian history, is it considered a holy plant? Some historians suggest that the blackberry was the burning bush in the story of Moses and the Ten Commandments.

Healthy eating devotees and lovers of blackberry pie may well ignore the myth and caution given the many health benefits of eating this special fruit.

Description of the Plant: common blackberry is an invasive shrub that grows up to five feet in height. Its distinguishing feature is its berry production, with very dark black fruit clusters which produce in mid-to late-summer. It has pinnately compound leaves with very prickly, stiff stems. Leaves are oblong to tapered, with toothed edges and prickles on the petioles.

Common Names: it is known as high bush blackberry and low bush blackberry.

How, When, and Where to Gather: blackberries commonly grow in the eastern USA and Canada, as well as the Pacific coast. They prefer temperate climates. Some types are found in every state and every province. In the past century, they have moved into the Midwest and are considered to be invasive. Their northern range is about 70 degrees north.

Blackberries prefer organic, well-drained soils, neutral to slightly acidic soil (pH 6.0-7.0), good sunlight, and moderate moisture. They will grow in almost any soil, however.

Blackberries produce fruit in early to mid-summer. Gathering berries in the early daytime will help them retain their moisture. If you are worried about brambles, use gloves when picking.

Health, Nutritional, and Medicinal Benefits: it is an antidiarrheal, anti-inflammatory, and also a diuretic.

Blackberry is viewed as a noxious weed by many, but has incredible health benefits due to its high nutrient content, antioxidant power, and stores of minerals and active chemical ingredients. It is used to treat diarrhea, whooping cough, cancer, dysentery, colitis, amenia, hemorrhoids, cancer, diabetes, gout, inflammation, toothache, sore throat, ulcers, and minor bleeding.

Edible Parts: You can eat both the fruit and the leaves.

Look-Alike Plants (Poisonous and Not): loganberries, boysenberries, and mulberries all are similar in appearance to blackberries. None are toxic and all are edible.

Recipe: Blackberry Rose Ice Pops

Ingredients

2 cup blackberries, washed and culled

½ cup rose petals, crushed

⅔ cup cane sugar

1 tablespoon lemon juice

Method:

Blend all ingredients in a blender until smooth. Pour into individual ice pop containers and freeze solid. Enjoy!

CHAPTER SIX:

BLUEBERRY

Latin Name: Vaccinium augustifolium

Try not to hum Fats Domino's tune of "I Found My Thrill on Blueberry Hill" now that it has been planted in your memory. Savor the taste of blueberries on ice cream or blueberries in sweet cream as you visualize the fruit. Then try to get your share of the fruit in the wild as you compete with bears, only months out of their winter sleep and still voracious. The fruit is hugely popular because of its wide availability, unique taste, memories of childhood foraging, and its health benefits.

A popular myth is that blueberries are the favorite fruit of angels, but they don't like the skins, so after a night of gorging on the fruit and tossing the skins aside, in the morning, the heavens are littered with these gorgeous blue skins, making the sky blue. They certainly make your tongue, fingers, and lips blue when they are eaten, but they are more than worth this inconvenience.

One of Robert Frost's longest poems deals with the virtues of blueberries. He talks of how others, picking in the same area where he was picking, look at him as if he has no right to share in their bounty.

Description of the Plant: the fruit is easily identified. Many of the plants grow low to the ground, but others grow as high as six feet, often in filtered sunlight at the edges of coniferous

59

woods. They frequently are found in the same area as bearberries. The flowers in spring start out as very small, teardrop-shaped buds developing into bell-shaped flowers. Leaves are ovate, with the oval wider at the bottom than the top and a toothed edge. Multiple stems grow from the long, branching roots each spring, with the roots often visible through the rotting leaves and mulch of the forest undergrowth.

Common Names: it is known as the huckleberry.

How, When, and Where to Gather: blueberries prefer acidic soil (4.2 to 5.2 pH), moderate moisture, and moderate to full sun. They grow primarily in the eastern two-thirds of the North American continent. Blueberries grow low to the ground and produce fruit in early summer. By mid-summer, berries begin to dry up, and wild animals, such as raccoons and bears, feast on them.

Health, Nutritional, and Medicinal Benefits: it is an anti-inflammatory, astringent, diuretic, antioxidant, anti-microbial, anti-edematous, venous tonic, vaso-protector, anti-platelet, antiemetic, and anti-diarrheal.

Blueberry is used to prevent cataracts and glaucoma. It treats ulcers, MS, fibromyalgia, urinary tract infections, fever, varicose veins, hemorrhoids, protects against heart disease, detoxifies the system, strengthens immunity, slows aging signs, prevents diabetes, stimulates circulation, and works as a laxative. Blueberries are very nutrient dense and very high in antioxidants.

Edible Parts: This bountiful berry is widely enjoyed and popular.

Look-Alike Plants (Poisonous and Not): salal, bilberries, pokeberries, nightshade, and buckthorn berries all resemble blueberries, but both pokeberries and nightshade are deadly poisonous to humans.

Recipe: **Wild blueberry Fruit Dip**

Ingredients

2 cups blueberries

1 cup whipped cream

1 cup plain cream cheese

¼ teaspoon nutmeg

Method:

Blend all ingredients together, but do not overdo it, let the berries remain relatively intact. Place in a decorative bowl and place other fruit like whole strawberries, large chunks of banana, apple, or pear slices around it to dip in.

CHAPTER SEVEN:
BURDOCK

Latin Name: Arctium lappa, Yellow Dock- Rumex crispus

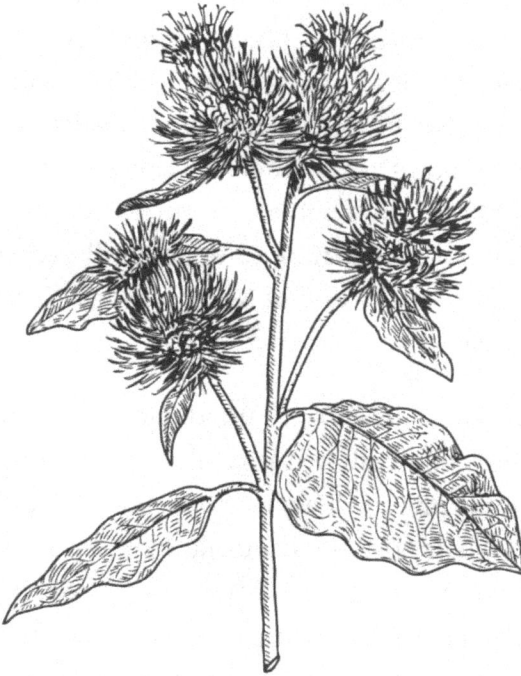

Late at night, pixies would amuse themselves by riding colts through the fields, planting horse's manes, which would become cockleburs. At least, that is the European myth.

In Greek mythology, burdock derives its feminine energy from the Greek goddess Venus. This "feminine energy" was credited with its blood cleansing powers and it often was used in folk medicine during and after pregnancy.

A young gardener tending a house that was on the market for sale, carefully mowed the grass around a plant near the entrance step, believing it to be either rhubarb or horseradish which he had seen often in local gardens. The plant, with its enormous leaves, grew over the next few months to nearly five feet tall, producing abundant leaves and small purplish flowers. The flowers were new to him, as were the seed pods that formed in late summer. They clung to him, attaching themselves painfully to his clothes, his hair, and even his skin. Instead of carefully tending a flower, he had been cultivating one of North America's most common weeds: burdock.

Description of the Plant: burdock may begin its life resembling horseradish, but its rapid growth quickly eclipses that of its look-alikes. The mature plant has an ungainly appearance, quite tall (exceeding five feet), with a thick, round, and woody stem and huge, shovel-sized leaves, up to eighteen inches long on multiple heavy branches. In the first year, it produces a handful of medium-sized leaves, growing in a rosette with a minimal stem. Its long, tapering root grows rapidly in that year. The young stems have numerous hairs, like cobwebs, but these hairs disappear in the second year, replaced by a veiny stalk.

Leaves look somewhat similar to horseradish or even very large rhubarb leaves, oblate in shape. They are dull green on top, facing the sun, and slightly whitened underneath.

The flowers do not emerge until the second year, appearing from July until frost comes. They are purple and are borne in small clustered heads with hooked spines. The spiny burs formed are great pests, attaching themselves to clothing and to the wool and hair of animals. The flowers appear somewhat similar to the purple flower of a thistle, with sheath bracts forming a cup around the flower, green at the base and yellowish-green toward the flower part. They have a spiny appearance. The flowers turn brown prior to forming seed pods that enclose the withered flower in late summer.

The plant has a large fleshy taproot. When dry, this root is much wrinkled lengthwise. Burdock is one of the easiest plants to find in the late fall and winter. Truthfully, you don't find burdock; it finds you, with its Velcro-inspired burs and tall, bush-like habit.

Common Names: it is known as cocklebur, cockle button, bardane, and bur.

How, When, and Where to Gather: burdock is not native to the Americas. Settlers from the old world introduced it to North America, and it now grows along roadsides and in fields and bush lines, near old homesteads, barnyards, pastures, and waste places. It is very abundant in the Eastern and Central States, all the Canadian provinces, and in many localities in the West, except the south-central United States.

It is extremely hardy and grows wherever animals have walked routinely. While it prefers nitrogen-rich soil, it will grow almost in any soil in full or partial sun. The roots form best in light well-drained soil.

Because the burs on the seed pod latch readily onto fur and clothes, the plant is spread widely. Once pets, for instance, gnaw the burs off their fur, the seed pod drops and grows where it falls, often near entrances, barns and buildings, underbrush where wild animals bed down, and so on. Stories abound that the inventor of Velcro used burs as the template for his invention.

Burdock roots can be harvested even in winter, since this tall weed often is visible above the snow. Leaves are best picked in early spring, before they become overly large and tough.

Edible Parts: young leaves and shoots, roots, occasionally seeds. In the spring of the plant's second year, harvest the roots and use them as a starch-like vegetable. They can be consumed fresh or sliced thin and dried. If you slice them too thick, the roots may become moldy quickly. You may harvest older roots in the fall and winter.

As a survival food in winter, burdock is a great cache. The plants are easy to find among snowdrifts, often towering above them. Chop the roots free of ice in colder regions and peel them, eaten raw or boiled. In spring the young, small leaves and early parts of the stems (peeled) are tender. They may be used in stews, soups, and salads, or sauteed with butter.

The flavor of burdock is a cross between sorrel and spinach with a bit of a tart tang. Because the leaves are high in oxalates (like rhubarb leaves and horseradish leaves), you should not consume large quantities at a time.

Burdock root and young stems may be peeled, sliced, lightly blanched, and stored in vinegar brine in the refrigerator for up to two weeks, producing a unique pickle.

The Japanese often use burdock, known as Gobo, in their culinary dishes.

Health, Nutritional, and Medicinal Benefits: burdock is an antioxidant, anti-inflammatory, stimulant, diuretic, laxative, antifungal, anticarcinogenic, antiviral, and antidiabetic.

Burdock has numerous medicinal uses and health benefits. Nutritionally, it is high in protein, beta carotene, Vitamin C, calcium, magnesium potassium, Vitamin E, folates, and zinc. It is used in liver cleanses, the leaves in poultices for skin damage and eruptions, the roots for hair and scalp treatments. Burdock has been used to treat colds and measles, relieve constipation, and purify the blood. Decoctions from the root and seeds, or infusions from the leaves are used to treat gout, colds, rheumatism, stomach ailments, cancer, and constipation.

Look-Alike Plants (Poisonous and Not): three plants that often get confused with burdock are primrose, foxglove, and rhubarb. Of the three, primrose and foxglove should be handled with care. Foxglove is the source of digitalis, a heart medication, but all parts of the plant are toxic. Primrose primarily grows in gardens in North America, but a variety of primrose–loosestrife is an invasive, noxious weed found around the continent. Primrose, like foxglove, is poisonous and causes serious skin irritation when touched.

The leaves may cause contact dermatitis for people with allergies. Some reports show that the leaves, when consumed in large quantities, can be toxic, because of its high oxalate content. Rhubarb, foxglove, primrose, and nightshades all have leaves similar to burdock, but foxglove, primrose, and nightshades are poisonous.

Recipe: **Burdock and Mushroom Brown Rice**

Ingredients

1 cup brown rice

2 cups water

1 shiitake mushroom, chopped

1 cup diced burdock root

4 garlic cloves

⅓ teaspoon ginger

Salt and pepper to taste

Method:

Cook brown rice, shiitake mushroom, burdock root, garlic, and ginger with the addition of salt and pepper to taste.

A great sauce recipe includes one cup burdock root, ½ cup parsley, ½ cup cider vinegar, ½ cup sherry, and one cup of thick yogurt (Greek, preferably). Boil the cider, burdock, and sherry over medium heat for six to eight minutes, then blend all ingredients until smooth. This sauce is fantastic with vegetables (particularly green veggies) pork or chicken.

CHAPTER EIGHT:

CATTAIL

Latin Name: Typha latifolia, Typha augustifolia

Of all the plants, cattail possibly has the most direct connection to religious lore and mythology. After all, it was in a bed of cattails, or bullrushes, that Egyptian royalty found the baby Moses. The rest is Christian history!

Early North American settlers relied on cattail seed pods as fire tinder, bedding and jacket insulation, and even insulation in shacks and shanties. They wove the leaves into baskets and even roofs of buildings and ate the roots and young leaves. The giant brown seed pod heads, soaked in coal oil or kerosene, acted as great torches. In marshes and ditches across wide swaths of the continent, cattails now are so prolific as to be considered a nuisance. Yet they are indispensable for our environment, filtering pollutants from entering major waterways. Their huge, Popsicle-shaped flower heads and seed pods are easily recognized.

Description of the Plant: the leaves–emerging from long, creeping rhizome roots–are long, thin, and somewhat tapered. The plant produces tiny, unisex flowers in a dense, cylinder-shaped head about four to six inches long. The flowers fall off after being pollinated, creating the brown, puffy knot that we readily recognize. Very late in the autumn and into the winter and spring, the brown, dense cylinder releases masses of cotton-tufted seeds, dispersed by the wind.

Cattails, or bullrushes, are one of the easiest plants in the marshes and waterways of North America to identify, and they are very abundant. Most people recognize the corn dog-shaped flower and seed head that sits atop the plant in the fall and winter, or the white fluff that erupts when the seed pod ripens and sends the seeds into the air. Almost as many recognize the tall (up to five feet), singular leaves, long, flat, and thin, that grow incredibly fast through the spring and summer. Few, though, see the light green shoots in the mud, or even under the water in early spring.

Common Names: it is known as broadleaf cattail, bulrush, common bulrush, and also as the common cattail.

How, When, and Where to Gather: cattails are one of the true survival foods of North America. Found in abundance throughout all North America, Mexico, and parts of the Caribbean islands, this versatile plant provides nourishment, shelter, flavoring, and heat.

It is not grown domestically, but can be planted successfully in decorative ponds. It grows best in heavy clay or sour soil in swamp edges and along slower creeks, drainage ditches, waterways, and even wastewater lagoons, where locals sometimes employ it as a "green filter" for domestic sewage. Cattails serve as this excellent natural filter in swamps at the heads of rivers and creeks leading to larger lakes, where nutrients are scooped out of the water mix by the plants, and larger waste trapped and consumed over time.

Health, Nutritional, and Medicinal Benefits: medicinally, cattails are hemostatic, astringent, diuretic, antiseptic, coagulant, and emmenagogue (aids in menstruation).

Cattails may be harvested throughout the year. Use plants harvested from clean water, as they pick up the toxins and pollutants from the surrounding soil and water. Nutritionally, cattails are high in fiber, sodium, calcium carbohydrates, manganese, vitamin K, and iron.

The young shoots in the spring are wonderful, raw or boiled, with a taste like borage or cucumber. The pollen from the flowers in the late spring makes a great thickener for various boiled dishes. The green buds that precede the small flowers are a great, crunchy snack in early summer. Throughout the year, roots are edible but, as they age, they pick up much of the pungent taste of the swampy water in which they grow.

The fibrous root network, when boiled, yields a great starchy paste that is great for "bread," or in soups. The root bulb itself tastes like a potato, and cooks like a potato, but can also be eaten raw. The roots may be dried and stored, as can the small flower head.

Use cattail pollen as an astringent and hemostatic, on cuts and wounds to control bleeding. Take it internally for chest pain and blood issues. Pounded root, as a poultice, is effective on wounds, bruises, and stings. Cattail has been used to treat anemia, cancer, diabetes, digestive disorders, hypertension, and hardening of the arteries.

Edible Parts: all parts of the cattail are used. As the plant reaches adulthood, leaves are no longer edible but remain useful.

Look-Alike Plants (Poisonous and Not): In the spring, when swamp, water and bog plants are young, species of Iris, Acorus, and some Bulrushes all resemble the young Cattail plants. Blue flag iris, which also grows in swampy areas in the United States, looks a lot like cattail but is poisonous. Any other look-alike is generally unpalatable, but not harmful. There are no known contraindications for Cattail. No adverse side effects or reactions have been documented with any consistency.

Recipe: Cattail Pancakes

Ingredients

½ cup flour

½ cup cattail pollen

1 cup dried cattail root flour

1 tsp baking powder

2 eggs

2 cups milk or water

½ cup honey

¼ cup oil

½ tsp vanilla or maple extract

Method:

Mix all dry ingredients. Lightly whisk eggs in a separate bowl, add in milk, honey, and vanilla, then blend wet and dry ingredients until a medium-thin paste forms. Cook like pancakes and serve with syrup and cinnamon.

CHAPTER NINE:

CHICKWEED

Latin Name: Stellaria media

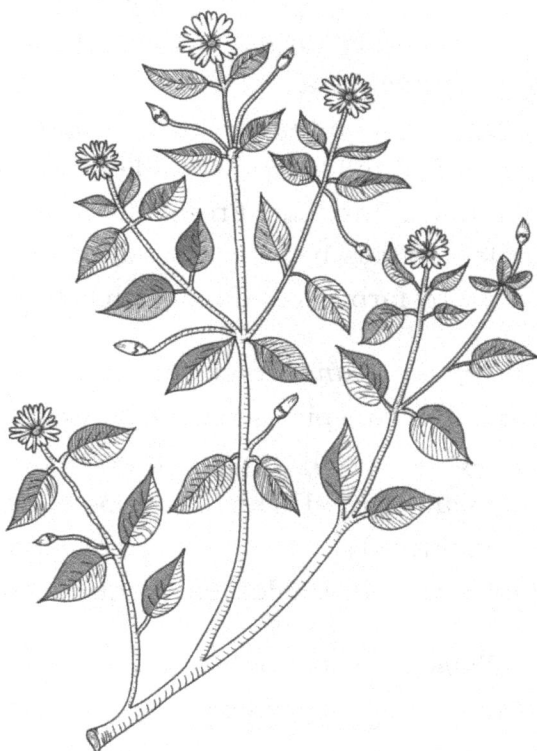

Chickweed–independent, sprawling, and free-ranging, is symbolic of family. In folklore, it is associated with balance, fidelity, and loyalty, yet it is a plant that loves its space. Between chickweed plants and among its own leaves, it spaces itself out, but grows in clusters in the same way that families and villages form bonds and rely on each other, yet give each other a bit of space.

The same plant to which hundreds of thousands of users are allergic and from which we experience hay fever symptoms has provided natural healing remedies for the First Nations of North America for centuries. Like goldenrod, it is a European plant, gone wild, naturalized to most of the continent, and adopted by indigenous people for both its nutritional and medicinal value. It was used for colds, whooping cough, bronchitis, and sore throats, and used as a fresh dietary "green" in late spring and early summer. Leaves are dried and made into teas. From a healthy dietary source for early settlers, it has become a scourge, considered to be a noxious weed by farmers and landscapers.

Description of the Plant: chickweed has small, bunched leaves and small, inconspicuous white flowers. It grows to 45 cm (18 in.), but generally hugs the ground, creeping and spreading. It is an annual. The leaves look similar to thyme leaves. It is considered a broadleaf weed because of the broad shape of the leaves, but the leaves are quite small.

Common Names: commonly called chickweed, field chickweed, and mouse ear chickweed.

How, When, and Where to Gather: common chickweed grows in most states, the coast and interior of British Columbia, Ontario, Quebec, the Maritime provinces, and southern portions of the prairie provinces. It is a noxious weed in many parts of the continent, invading lawns and fields. It is a Eurasian plant that now is naturalized in most of North America, preferring fields and lawns (bright sun to partial shade), moist and loamy soils. Pick in early spring when both leaves and stems are still tender. Later in the spring and summer, pick only the leaves and flowers.

Health, Nutritional, and Medicinal Benefits: chickweed is a demulcent, anti-inflammatory, and anti-irritation.

Chickweed contains phytosterols, tocopherols, triterpene saponins, flavonoids, and Vitamin C. Consuming excessive amounts of chickweed can cause nausea, upset stomach, and diarrhea.

Chickweed is used to treat itches and skin conditions. It also is used to treat pulmonary diseases, iron deficiency, bronchitis, arthritis, and menstrual period pain. It can be used as an eyewash. Chickweed may relieve constipation, stomach and bowel problems, blood disorders, asthma and other lung diseases, obesity, scurvy, psoriasis, itching, and muscle or joint pain. Chickweed supports digestion and weight loss and heals wounds.

Blend in a blender, ½ cup chickweed leaves, and ¼ cup carrier oil like olive or almond oil to use and apply topically.

Edible Parts: you can eat the leaves, flowers, and stems. Chickweed leaves go well in fresh salads, soups, and egg recipes.

Look-Alike Plants (Poisonous and Not): a toxic look-alike is the scarlet pimpernel. However, the scarlet pimpernel has reddish-brown flowers rather than white.

Recipe: **Chickweed Pesto**

Ingredients

½ cup walnuts

3 cloves garlic

3 cups chickweed leaves, packed

1 tbsp lemon juice

½ cup grapeseed oil

½ tsp salt

¼ cup parmesan cheese

Salt and pepper to taste

Method:

Blend in a blender until smooth and refrigerate.

CHAPTER TEN:
CHICORY

Latin Name: Cichorium intybus

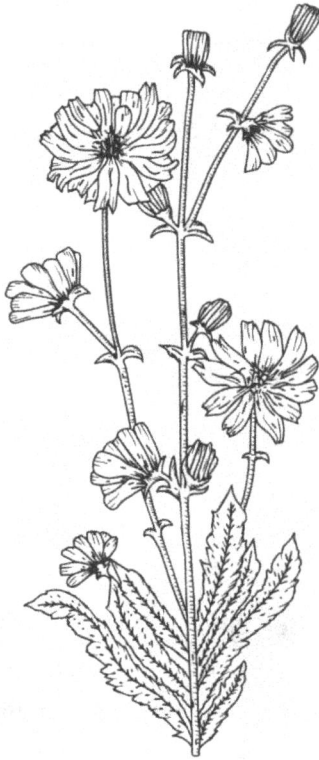

Chicory is associated with Clytie, Apollo's illicit lover. Tales of her exploits, as she would engage in a secret triste each morning with Apollo, spring from Chicory's habit of blooming only in the early morning hours.

Chicory may be one of the essential wilderness survival foods if one needs a cup of java each morning. While the taste of ground chicory coffee is nothing like real coffee, it does offer a bitter stop-gap substitute and, at least, a perceived jolt of energy. Chicory contains no caffeine, but it has a much higher soluble content than coffee, giving it that essential strong kick.

Classic Western movies always seem to have cowboys drinking coffee every morning on a roundup, but it is more likely that they were using chicory or dandelion root, ground and boiled. Chicory only blooms in the early morning, making it easily identified for wanderers seeking their morning beverage.

For the devout, religious symbolism places Chicory as a bitter symbol of Christ's passion.

Description of the Plant: Chicory roots are long and fleshy taproots. The stem is rigid, branching, and hairy, growing up to five feet, but more commonly under three feet. Leaves are lobed and toothed, looking somewhat like dandelion leaves. They grow around the base. Flowers are blue and sometimes white. The plant begins as a rosette in the spring as the stems emerge from the root base. Later in the spring and early summer, one stem emerges from the rosette, growing to the plant's full height as it produces flowers from the stem.

Common Names: known as blue daisy, cornflower, wild endive, and wild bachelor's buttons.

How, When, and Where to Gather: Chicory can be found in abandoned fields, areas along roads and rails, untended grassy areas, undeveloped land, waste areas, and pastures. These are the same locales where both hawthorn and horseradish—two plants introduced to North America by Europeans—also thrive. That is, they often are found near old homesteads and living areas of early settlers. It likes limestone and gravelly soils. Chicory roots can be harvested in spring, summer, and fall. In the fall, the essential oils focus in the roots, giving them a strong taste. Chicory buds produce in late spring.

Chicory is found throughout North America, growing west to California, and south to Florida.

Health, Nutritional, and Medicinal Benefits: it is trophorestorative, emollient, laxative, demulcent, refrigerant, and anti-inflammatory.

Although chicory commonly is associated with being a coffee substitute on trail rides, its medicinal properties go well beyond that. It is an appetite stimulant, tonic for urine output, liver protector, and used to balance the stimulant effect of coffee. It also treats gallstones, sinus problems, constipation, liver issues, cancer, rapid heartbeat, and gastroenteritis. Externally, it can be applied to cuts and bruises, and used to help reduce swelling and inflammation.

Edible Parts: you can eat the root, leaves, and the buds.

Look-Alike Plants (Poisonous and Not): there are no poisonous plants that are confused with chicory, making them, along with dandelion, the safest plants to harvest in the wild.

Recipe: **Sauteed Chicory**

Ingredients

1 bunch chicory leaves, washed

2 cloves crushed garlic

¼ teaspoon red pepper flakes

¼ teaspoon turmeric

salt to taste

2 tablespoons butter or olive oil

¼ cup sunflower seeds, shelled and cooked

Method:

Sauté ingredients in butter for three to four minutes, or until tender. Serve, sprinkle with shredded mozzarella cheese or three tablespoons of plain Greek yogurt mixed with one tablespoon of lemon juice.

Chapter Eleven:
Dandelion

Latin Name: Taraxacum officianale

You face a choice: eradicate them or enjoy them. Every spring, almost the first flower to bloom in the northern hemisphere seems to be dandelions, across every lawn north of the 49th parallel, and even well down into the south-central United States. Europe, too, has dandelions in abundance.

Dandelions have a spiritual meaning, too. They represent hope, light, and healing. They denote strength, peace, growth, happiness, and playfulness. But still, they are walked on, sprayed and eradicated, and loathed. Yet, in an odd irony, young hearts wherever the plant grows, puff on the seed pods and make a wish, hopeful for the future. It is this love/hate relationship that is at the heart of the need to eliminate them while also making use of every part of the plant to sustain us and keep us healthy.

But dandelions are only noxious weeds because of our perception of them. In fact, they are one of the best sources of nourishment in any plant, from flower to root. They arrived in North America as a garden flower, cultivated in Europe.

In the spring, the young dandelion greens (the tender leaves) are delicious in salads or boiled and buttered, with thyme.

Dandelion easily is one of the most versatile nutritional and medicinal plants that can be harvested in the wild in North America. Root, leaves, and flowers of the dandelion all can be consumed, for both health benefits and culinary uses.

Description of the Plant: imagine a small version of the sunflower without the dark center of florets. The dandelion flower is one of the most recognizable wild flowers in North America, with its bright yellow face of petals. It grows across all of North America, but does particularly well in colder northern climates. It is one of the first northern latitude flowers to bloom in spring, after crocuses and marsh marigolds, but can bloom all year if it keeps being cut by mowers or eaten by livestock. The flowers reappear days after the previous flower is cut, often on shorter milk-filled stems than the prior one. The leaves form at the base of the plant. They are toothed, but the teeth usually are smooth.

Common Names: It is known as bitter wort, Irish daisy, and clock flower.

How, When, and Where to Gather: harvest dandelion leaves in early spring, before they become mature, tough, and bitter. The flowers are harvested throughout their blooming period. The roots are best harvested in early and late summer.

Health, Nutritional, and Medicinal Benefits: it is a diuretic, choleretic, anti-inflammatory, cholagogue, tonic, antirheumatic, bitter, alterative, and depurative.

Dandelion is used as a tonic, blood purifier, gallbladder, kidney, and urinary tract disorder treatment, liver treatment for jaundice and hepatitis, to relieve constipation, as a salve for inflammatory skin conditions, joint pain, and eczema. It also is used to treat hypoglycemia, edema associated with high blood pressure, gout, and even acne.

Edible Parts: You can eat the roots, young leaves, and flowers (make wine).

Look-Alike Plants (Poisonous and Not): None.

Recipe: **Dandelion Bean Skillet**

Ingredients

2 bunches washed dandelion greens

¼ sliced red onion

2 cloves garlic, crushed

1 teaspoon oregano

¼ teaspoon black pepper

2 cans fava or kidney beans

½ cup peanuts

Method:

Sauté onion and garlic in two tablespoons of butter or olive oil until tender then add remaining ingredients, season with salt and pepper, and serve.

CHAPTER TWELVE:
FIELD MUSTARD

Latin Name: Allaria petiolata, Brassica juncea

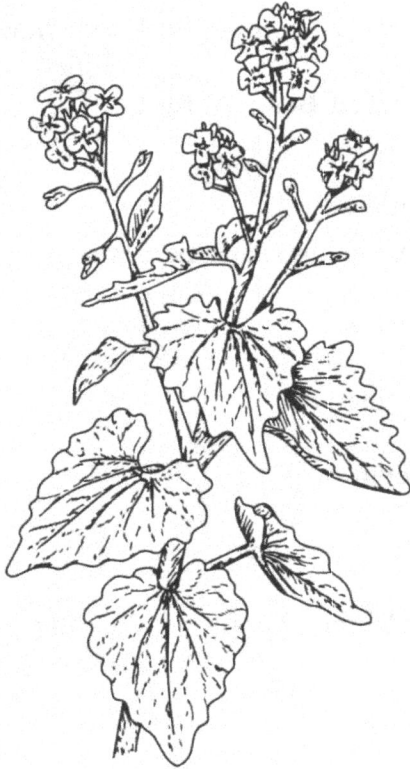

The tiny mustard seed finds itself at the center of several of Christ's parables about faith. Mohammed's teachings focus on faith, describing the value in the smallest amount of faith as "even as tiny as the tiny mustard seed" as immeasurably important. Yet, mustard finds itself eschewed by many, criticized for the potential it has in the way of digestive harm, often discarded as waste, and reviled as a weed by farmers.

A group exploring the potential to use different feedstocks—sources of oil—for a local biodiesel plant hit upon the idea of using the waste from seed cleaning facilities in the area. Most of the waste seed that the cleaners screened from the grain and canola crops was wild mustard. It contained between 35-45 percent oil that was quite suitable for biodiesel.

This oil, being "hot" and high in uric acid, harmed the digestive system so the mustard seed could not be found in the waste byproducts of biodiesel that often were fed to cattle. However, the farmers discovered that the paste remaining from the extraction process, spread around the perimeter of gardens, worked wonders at repelling crawling insects and small rodents. They used practical applications, instead of the religious faith surrounding the mustard seed in the Bible, Hinduism, Islam, and Buddhism.

Description of the Plant: Mustard starts out as a basal plant with rosettes springing from the root. Flowering stems do not emerge until the second year. Plants grow up to four feet tall with a multi-branched stem. The leaves often develop a white color later in summer. Lower leaves are rough-shaped, a little like small rhubarb or burdock leaves, and about a foot long with up to four lobes. Upper leaves have no lobes. Flowers are yellow and look similar to tansy flowers, clumped in a small head.

Common Names: it is known as wild turnip and wild kale.

How, When, and Where to Gather: Field mustard loves sandy and clay soils and has a wide pH range of 4.8 to 8.5. It grows in most disturbed areas, as well as gardens and fields, invading crops like canola. It can be found along roads, in ditches, in orchards, and even in unmowed lawns. It is considered a noxious weed because of its adaptability. It has spread to almost all of the North American continent. Harvest leaves in early spring, before the heat of summer makes them tough and harsh-tasting. The seeds are ready in late July and August.

Health, Nutritional, and Medicinal Benefits: it is an antirheumatic, anti-bronchial, irritant, stimulant, diuretic, and emetic.

For many people, mustard poultices come with memories of childhood, as the hot patches on the chest relieved coughs and colds effectively. For others, it was an anti-worm treatment. Wild mustard has the same, only more intense, qualities as domestic yellow mustard. It opens blood vessels, allowing the system to detoxify and increase blood flow. It reduces pain and swelling. It is effective as a headache treatment when consumed as tea. Mustard is also used to treat painful joints and muscles, arthritis, relieving edema, increasing urine output, and increasing appetite.

Mustard can be used to treat painful joints and muscles, relieve arthritis and edema, increase urine output, and increase appetite.

Edible Parts: You can eat the young leaves, seeds (spice), and the flowers.

Look-Alike Plants (Poisonous and Not): Wild mustard and wild rapeseed or canola look like mustard, but none of these are poisonous.

Recipe: Stir-Fried Chinese Mustard Greens

Ingredients

1 ½ pounds mustard greens

¼ cup crushed almonds

4 cloves garlic

½ teaspoon red pepper flakes

½ teaspoon Chinese Five Spice

½ pound bok choy

1 ½ teaspoons cane sugar

2 teaspoons sesame oil

1 teaspoon lemon juice

Method:

Add garlic and chili to two tablespoons of hot oil in a wok. Cook for one minute, add mustard greens, and bok choy. Cook for two minutes, then add remaining ingredients, season with salt and pepper, and cook for another two minutes, tossing as it cooks.

CHAPTER THIRTEEN:
JERUSALEM ARTICHOKE

Latin Name: Helianthus tuberosus

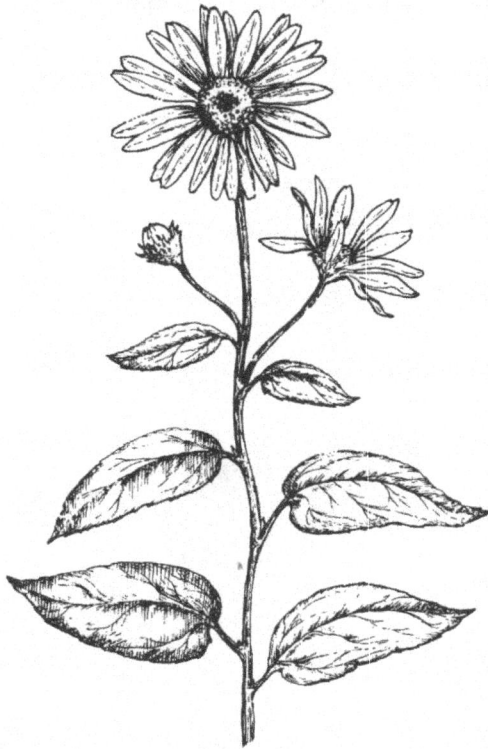

Jerusalem artichoke has an ugly, unpleasant lore associated with it, playing on the ignorant prejudices of people of the Middle Ages. Because of its gnarled root, it was shunned as the plant of lepers, its twisted shapes mimicking the deformities of people with the disease.

For those wildcrafters who believe they are searching after an artichoke when they head out to harvest the Jerusalem artichoke, nothing could be further from the truth. The Jerusalem artichoke is not an artichoke and is not from Jerusalem. In fact, it is a sunflower that is grown not for its sunflower or seeds, but for its tuberous root.

The name appears to come from a British corruption of the word *girasol*, meaning "sunflower," then adding the word "artichoke" because of its taste, similar to an artichoke.

Everything about the Jerusalem artichoke is peculiar. It was, at one time, an important root crop export from North America and was known as the 'Canada potato', even though the range for this tuber is very limited in Canada but spreads across the entire United States. Even though it was sometimes called the leprosy potato because of its appearance similar to the gnarled digits of a leper and was shunned by many, it continued to grow in popularity. This plant was originally not found anywhere except in North America but now is one of the most commonly cultivated garden plants in all of Europe.

Description of the Plant: Jerusalem Artichoke has many characteristics in common with the rest of the sunflower family. It grows two to eight feet tall, with the occasional stem branches in the top half of its length. Stems are light green, hairy, and pithy. Leaves are opposite on the lower half of the plant, alternate toward the top, with a rough, hairy texture. The leaves also are larger on the bottom and are the typical sunflower-shaped broad, ovate-acute, while at the top they are smaller, narrower, and less abundant. The flowers look the same as most sunflowers, but smaller—roughly half the size of a sunflower. Briefly, these flowers emit a lovely chocolate-vanilla scent as they attract pollinators.

Common names: they are known as sunchokes, earth apples, and sunroots.

How, When, and Where to Gather: Jerusalem artichoke comes from the eastern United States, where it was a significant food crop for native American tribes. It now grows in every state except Arizona, New Mexico, Nevada, Alaska, Hawaii, and every Canadian province east of Saskatchewan. It prefers moist meadows and valleys, and is common in old gardens and homesteads, fence lines, and roadsides. Roots reach maturity in late summer. Smaller leaves can be consumed throughout the growing period, as can the stalks.

Health, Nutritional, and Medicinal Benefits: it is an antioxidant, antidiabetic, anti-carcinogenic, anti-fungistatic, and anti-constipation remedy.

The root, stem, and leaves have many medicinal and health applications along with their culinary use. It has lots of iron, potassium, and Vitamin B1. They are gut healthy, a source of probiotics, inulin, and fiber. Jerusalem artichoke helps to fight obesity, helps the immune system, works well with insulin, modulates metabolism, and helps muscle function.

Edible Parts: you can eat the root and small leaves (shredded for salads).

Look-Alike Plants (Poisonous and Not): many other members of the sunflower look like Jerusalem artichoke, but none are toxic.

Recipe: **Roasted Jerusalem Artichoke**

Ingredients

1 pound Jerusalem artichoke root

½ cup avocado oil

salt and pepper to taste

2 tablespoons oregano or marjoram

¾ tablespoon powdered garlic

Method:

Set the oven to 350° Fahrenheit. Peel, trim, and clean the root, cutting it into one-inch pieces. Toss all the ingredients together in a large bowl. Place root on an open roasting pan or cookie sheet and bake in the oven for 45 minutes, turning occasionally, and drizzling spiced liquid on roots.

CHAPTER FOURTEEN:
LAMB'S QUARTERS

Latin Name: Chenopodium album

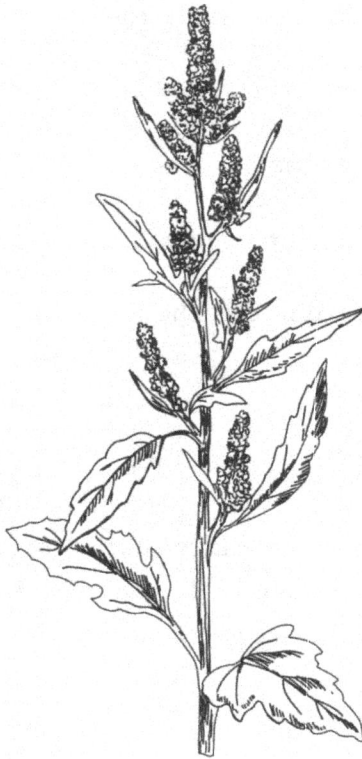

Lamb's quarters is a symbol and plant of immortality in Greek mythology where many healing plants find their history.

Lamb's quarters is a somewhat more romantic name than its other names, pigweed or goosefoot. Lamb's Quarters has been mostly shunned by the modern world, but not so in indigenous cultures. It is an ungainly plant that, supposedly, even pigs reluctantly ate. Yet, many families familiar with its taste, abundance, and nutritional value consumed it in the 1900s as a staple part of the summer diet. It ranks right up there with ragweed as a less-than-attractive dish.

Indigenous people in western Canada introduced settlers to pigweed as a staple food. Even though it has a very short growing season and is a very leggy plant with lots of stems, the First Nations people knew it was good for health and good for meals. Settlers, within the confines of a barracks or fort, rejected the plant as only worthy of being fed to the pigs, and some claimed that even the pigs rejected it. Of course it is not true, but it was part of the practice of denigrating anything associated with the indigenous people as being "savage" and unworthy.

Description of the Plant: lamb's quarters, or sometimes called pigweed, can grow up to six feet tall, but generally grow to about three feet. There also is a prostrate species of pigweed that is very edible. Leaves are pinnate, alternately arranged, small, narrow at the base, and waxy. The flower head is conical, growing from the center of the plant. The stem is round with ridges running vertically.

Common Names: known as goosefoot, pigweed, and also wild spinach.

How, When, and Where to Gather: lamb's quarters loves cultivated fields and crops, gardens, waste areas, roadsides and ditches, riverbanks, and other disturbed soils. They are native to North America. They tolerate most soils but have an affinity for nutrient-rich soils. They are listed as noxious weeds in many states and provinces. Pick the leaves in spring and early summer. Stems become woody as the summer progresses.

Health, Nutritional, and Medicinal Benefits: it is useful as an anti-anemic, astringent, antispasmodic, hepatoprotective, laxative, vulnerary, anti-inflammatory, analgesic, anthelmintic, and antimicrobial.

While lamb's quarters often is used in soups or salads, due to its high Vitamin A and C content as well as folate and calcium, it has many medicinal uses in folklore. These include treatments to alleviate fever, nausea, headache, stomach ache, sore throat, diarrhea, internal ulcers, and even menstrual bleeding. It has been linked topically to folk treatments for tumors, warts, and sores.

Edible Parts: you can eat the leaves, flowers, and stems.

Look-Alike Plants (Poisonous and Not): Lamb's Quarters are in the amaranth family, and look similar to many other wild-growing species of that family. No toxic look-alikes are known.

Recipe: **Lamb's Quarters Soup**

Ingredients

3 pounds chicken wings

1 quart chicken broth

½ pulped avocado

2 teaspoons oregano

1 red onion sliced thin

3 stalks celery, chopped,

2 pounds lamb's quarters

1 teaspoon seasoning salt

½ teaspoon black pepper

2 teaspoons crushed garlic

1 teaspoon paprika or cumin

Method:

In a slow cooker, add chicken broth, wings, and two cups of water. Simmer for ten to fifteen minutes, then add avocado, oregano, onion, celery, paprika, garlic, and salt. Simmer for another hour, until meat falls from the bones. Remove bones and strain mix to make sure no fragments of bone remain. Return to the crockpot, add lamb's quarters, and cook for five minutes.

CHAPTER FIFTEEN:
MILKWEED

Latin Name: Asclepias tuberosa, Asclepias syriaca

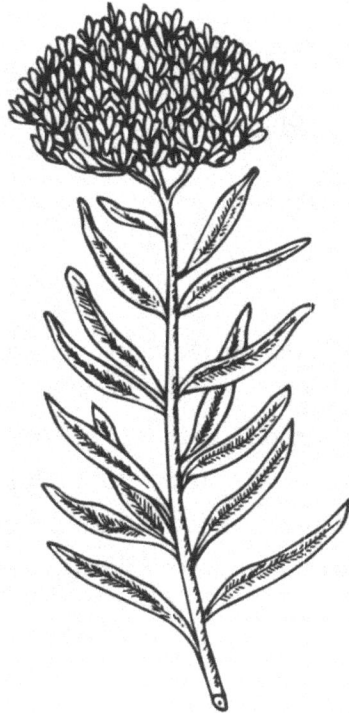

In Greek mythology, milkweed was Asclepios' gift from Apollo, a plant that is vital to curing external wounds. Asclepios, the son of Apollo, was recognized as the god of healing. Yet, milkweed is considered to be quite toxic to humans. Perhaps it is because of Apollo's reputation as a cunning god that this dichotomy between healing and destruction is found in one plant.

If only for its value to the monarch butterfly population, milkweed is a treasured plant. For the past century, farmers have viewed milkweed as a scourge of their crops, devoting intense efforts to eradicating this plant through the use of airborne chemicals and systemic herbicides.

But monarch butterflies only lay their eggs on milkweed and, without the plant, the monarch butterfly would become extinct. Still, huge swaths of farmland across the entire migratory path of the monarch butterfly no longer have milkweed, and the population of these beautiful insects is dropping precipitously.

Now, recognizing the peril to the only migratory butterfly in North America, gardeners and biologists are planting milkweed, hoping to assist the butterfly's recovery.

And, although milkweed is potentially poisonous to humans, it has wonderful medicinal properties when applied topically.

Description of the Plant: Milkweed grows to about five feet in height, but most commonly to about three feet. The leaves have a heavy, leathery look to them, are elongated oval and medium size, with a prominent midrib and tapered distal point. There usually are clusters of stout stems. Both leaves and stems exude a milky substance when broken. Flowers typically are in clusters. Leaves are the opposite. Flowers have five separate petals and five fused petals. They are greenish-pink to light purple. Seed pods are borne by the wind on dandelion-like tufts.

Common Names: it is also known as butterfly flower and silkweed.

How, When, and Where to Gather: milkweed, the mainstay for monarch butterflies, grows along the migration path of these insects in Canada and the United States. Only the west coast does not see a population of milkweed. Milkweed likes fence rows, roadsides, and garden edges, but does not cultivate well. It often is found in field crops, prairies, and pastures. It has been targeted by systemic and aerial applications of herbicides due to its invasive nature in grain crops. This has contributed to a decline in Monarch populations in the grain belts. Pick the young leaves and shoots in early to mid-spring.

Health, Nutritional, and Medicinal Benefits: emetic, diuretic, anthelmintic, stomachic, antidiarrheal, and diuretic.

While milkweed commonly is thought of as the Monarch butterfly's egg-laying station or as a noxious weed by farmers, it has medicinal value both externally and internally. It is potentially poisonous when overused, but, externally, it is an effective treatment for warts, to treat swelling, rashes, ringworm, boils, wounds, headache, skin ulcers, and skin lesions. Internally, it has been used by native Americans to treat snakebite, respiratory ailments, heart conditions, gas and diarrhea, pneumonia, and lung inflammation.

Edible Parts: the young shoots and leaves can be eaten (boiled, cooked).

Look-Alike Plants (Poisonous and Not): dogbane and milkweed look similar before they flower, but milkweed can be mildly toxic if consumed. Purple loosestrife looks vaguely similar to milkweed, but it grows in different habitats.

Recipe: Almond-Fried Milkweed Pods

Ingredients

4 oz. milkweed seed pods

1 cup buttermilk

salt to taste

¼ teaspoon cayenne pepper

½ teaspoon ground nutmeg

½ cup almond flour

¼ cup crushed cereal, like Cheerios or similar

Method:

Blanch the milkweed pods in boiling water for two to four minutes. Remove, drain, and cool. Soak pods in buttermilk for one to two hours. Mix remaining ingredients in a bowl, remove pods from buttermilk, and drain. Toss in the spice mix and fry in avocado oil or grapeseed oil until the pods are golden brown.

CHAPTER SIXTEEN:
MINER'S LETTUCE

Latin Name: Claytonia perfoliata

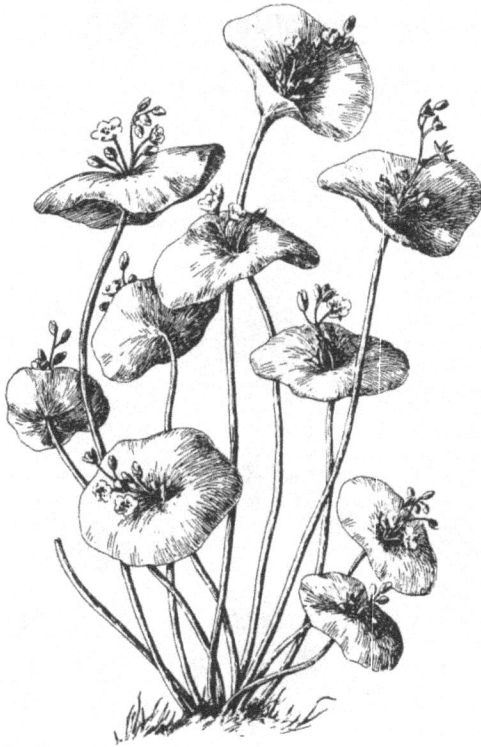

Sometimes a name reveals the folklore behind a plant. Miner's lettuce is one such plant. Its name comes from its use as a salad ingredient for miners in the western states and British Columbia, where it was one of the first greens to emerge in the spring. Its coarse nature reminds you that it, like rhubarb and burdock leaves, is prone to accumulating oxalates which can be toxic when consumed in large quantities.

Yet, prior to its adoption by the miners of the Pacific mountains, indigenous Americans already had embraced the plant, endowing it with mythical powers. To inject it with the formic acid from ant bites, they placed the plants on ant hills prior to consuming them, looking to capture the sting of the ant before heading out to hunt or fight. Like many aspects of their lives, North American Indians felt that the gods of the Earth were found in everything around them.

Description of the Plant: the leaves of miner's lettuce look similar to those of nasturtium, only smaller. They are almost disc-shaped, and less than an inch across. Leaves are borne on thin stems that have a slightly peppery taste. The plant grows low to the ground with immature stems. Flowers grow from what appears to be the center of the leaf and are very small and white.

Common Names: it is also called winter purslane and "Indian lettuce".

How, When, and Where to Gather: miner's lettuce grows mostly along the west coast and northern Mexico, as far east as Wyoming and Alberta. Being a cool-season, early spring plant, it prefers the altitudes of the foothills and medium elevations, but its season is short. It is most abundant in California and Oregon. Miner's lettuce, being a cool-weather crop, is only suitable for picking in early to mid-spring.

Health, Nutritional, and Medicinal Benefits: it is used as an antioxidant, laxative, diuretic, and also antirheumatic.

Although Miner's lettuce is popular as a salad green, and is high in Vitamin C and antioxidants, it also works as an appetite restorer, a laxative, general tonic, a blood purifier, and liver detoxifier. Use it in a poultice to treat rheumatic pain.

Edible Parts: you can eat the blossoms, stems, and leaves.

Look-Alike Plants (Poisonous and Not): dollar weed is a toxic look-alike of miner's lettuce, but it is not as common.

Recipe: Beet & Miner's Lettuce Salad

Ingredients

2 cups washed miner's lettuce leaves

1 cup coarsely diced, cooked, or pickled beets

1 cup mixed citrus fruit, chopped into quarter-sized pieces

½ cup plain or flavored yogurt

½ teaspoon cinnamon

1 tablespoon cane sugar

2 tablespoons vinaigrette dressing

Method:

Mix all ingredients except cinnamon and cane sugar. Sprinkle the last two ingredients on top of the salad right before serving.

Chapter Seventeen:
Nipplewort

Latin name: Lapsana communis

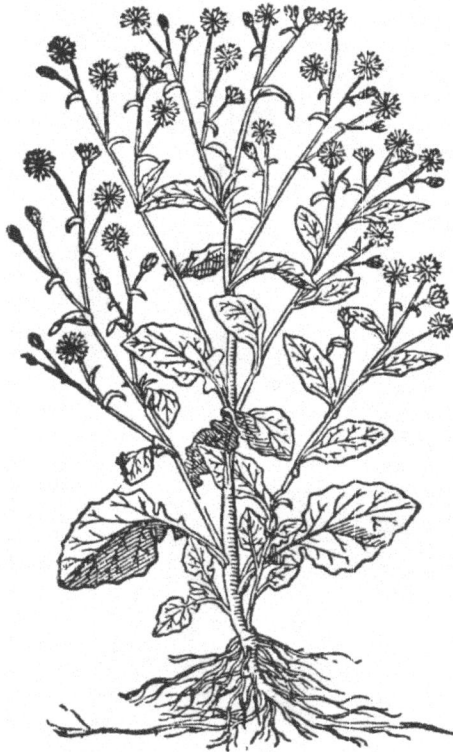

While "nipplewort" may seem to be an awkward common name for a plant, one of its other names, "Pilewort," is even more cringe-worthy. This is the lesser celandine, a delicately-flowered plant with blooms like its cousin, the buttercup, that look like the sun on a stem.

Although it has a long pedigree of curing a range of ailments, its mythological reputation as a source of joy and cure for depression is more in keeping with its bright appearance.

Nipplewort gets its name from its application to induce cows to provide more milk, while the pilewort's moniker is from, of course, its use as a treatment for hemorrhoids.

Description of the Plant: because it is a member of the sunflower family, it has many similar characteristics, including the sunflower or aster style of flower, with yellow petals in a circle around a collection of smaller florets (up to 700). When the plant emerges in the spring, it will have a bouquet look to it, with a rosette of leaves with one large terminal lobe and several smaller ones below. Then, the plant will bolt from its center, like a spinach plant bolting in the heat. Flowering occurs mid to late summer. Leaves are slightly toothed and rounded, thin and ovulate, pinnated. They look like small versions of an oak leaf, but the edges are somewhat serrated.

Common Names: it is also called the western rattlesnake root, wall lettuce, yellow spit, and even swallow wort.

How, When, and Where to Gather: nipplewort grows well in moist, shaded areas. Nipplewort is found in woods, fields, and disturbed sites like abandoned homesteads. It grows in much of temperate North America, and is more common in humid areas. Pick the shoots in spring and the leaves no later than early summer.

Health, Nutritional, and Medicinal Benefits: it is antiseptic and calming.

Nipplewort, as the name crudely suggests, is used to staunch the flow of breast milk. It also is used as a calming agent, helps with urinary tract infections, and treats kidney disease.

Edible Parts: you can eat the leaves and the shoots.

Look-Alike Plants (Poisonous and Not): there are no true look-alikes of this plant, but its flowers closely resemble dandelion flowers.

Recipe: **Nipplewort and Butternut BBQ Fry**

Ingredients

2 cups butternut squash

1 teaspoon nutmeg

salt and pepper to taste

2 cups nipplewort leaves, washed and blanched

¼ cup butter, cubed

¼ cup olive oil

Method:

Cube squash into one-inch cubes. Mix with nutmeg, salt, pepper, nipplewort, and butter. Pour into a loaf pan or heavy foil "boat." Add olive oil and seal with foil. Barbeque for twenty minutes, turning occasionally. Uncover for five minutes to sear squash.

CHAPTER EIGHTEEN:
PLANTAIN

Latin Name: Plantago major

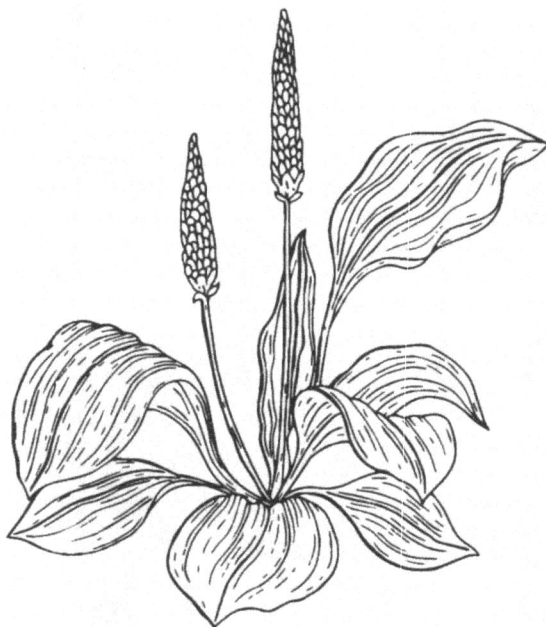

While many herbs have strong associations with religion, mythology, or even witchcraft, the poor, trod-upon, overlooked common plantain only manages brief references in witches' brews and Wiccan beliefs, and that is as a beneficial plant. Its only other common name in witchcraft is white man's foot. The name comes, not from its appearance, but from the general neglect of people who crush the plant underfoot.

Description of the Plant: common plantain is easily distinguished, after the first time you identify it. The leaves are broad and medium to dark green with prominent veins. The plant forms basal rosettes of these leaves and the plant rarely exceeds a few inches in height. In the late summer, the green flower spike forms, followed by seeds along this three or four-inch stem. The seeds turn brown as autumn arrives.

Common Names: it is known as broadleaf plantain and common plantain.

How, When, and Where to Gather: common plantain leaves reach maturity in mid-summer. They start later in the spring. They can be harvested throughout the growing season, but the seeds are not ready until late summer and early autumn. Find them wherever the soil has been disturbed, in fields and gardens, along pathways where people walk often, along roadsides, in gravelly, marginal soil to rich, well-drained soil.

Health, Nutritional, and Medicinal Benefits: tonic, emollient, anticatarrhal, vulnerary, expectorant, anti-inflammatory, refrigerant, diuretic, deobstruent, and antibacterial.

The leaves form excellent bandages on wounds, healing and protecting them. Plantain is an effective topical treatment for cuts, bites and stings, rashes, and bruises. It is used for treating coughs, inflammation, and infections. It also is used to treat burns, ulcers, and urinary tract infections.

Edible Parts: you can eat the leaves and the seeds (psyllium). Common plantain leaves are used in soups and stews, and very young leaves are used in salads, but have a texture like kale. The seeds (psyllium) are used as thickeners in soups and a partial substitute for starch.

Look-Alike Plants (Poisonous and Not): there are almost no look-alikes for the very distinctive common plantain. The closest that grows in a similar habitat and range would be the young sow thistle, but it grows much taller. Some varieties of plantain species also exist across North America.

Recipe: **Broadleaf Plantain Chips**

Ingredients

3 cups washed plantain leaves

salt to taste

sesame oil

Method:

Blanch plantain leaves for three to five minutes, scatter on an oven or air fryer wire rack to drain, and spread leaves out as much as possible without breaking them. Spritz them with sesame oil and sprinkle salt over the top. Cook at 400°F in an air fryer for eight minutes, or in the oven at 325°F for fifteen to twenty minutes until the leaves are crisp and curled.

CHAPTER NINETEEN:
PURSLANE

Latin Name: Portulaca oleracea

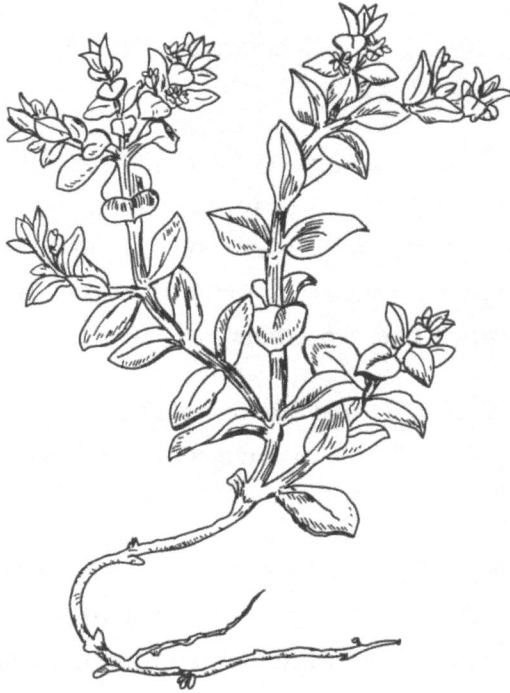

In ancient times, purslane, or wild portulaca, was scattered around a bed to protect against evil spirits. It falls under the influence of the moon, and is associated with the Greek goddesses Phoebe and Aramis, and the Roman goddess Diana.

Description of the Plant: purslane grows low to the ground on immature stems that look more like vines. Leaves are small and succulent, thick-looking, green, and oval in shape. Stems are reddish in color. The flowers are small and yellow. It is an annual that grows like a mat or carpet. It is considered invasive in many states and provinces and can be difficult to eradicate in rich soils. It is found around the world in temperate climates.

Common Names: it is known as little hogweed and wild portulaca.

How, When, and Where to Gather: purslane grows in full sun in almost any soil and invades lawns, gardens, and field crops easily. Purslane leaves should be harvested in late spring and early summer, along with flower buds. The seeds in late summer have a peppery taste.

Health, Nutritional, and Medicinal Benefits: it is a purgative, cardiac tonic, emollient, muscle relaxant, anti-inflammatory, and diuretic.

Although it is considered a weed, purslane has many medicinal and nutritional uses. It is used to treat burns, intestinal problems, headaches, liver issues, cough, arthritis, blood health, and diabetes. It is exceptionally high in Omega-3. It can help prevent stroke and heart disease.

Edible Parts: you can eat the leaves, flower buds, and stems.

Look-Alike Plants (Poisonous and Not): spurge, another noxious weed, looks very similar to purslane but is poisonous. Spurge stems are not as thick, and the leaves are smaller and not succulent in appearance.

Recipe: Tomato, Cucumber, and Purslane Salad

Ingredients

1 cucumber, peeled, sliced, and slices halved

2 medium tomatoes, chopped into ½ inch bites

1 bunch purslane, coarsely chopped

1-2 tablespoons fresh oregano, chopped

1 tablespoon lemon juice

¼ cup plain yogurt

2 teaspoons cane sugar

Method:

Mix cucumber, tomato, and purslane in a bowl. Blend lemon juice, yogurt, oregano, and sugar. Pour over salad vegetables and serve.

CHAPTER TWENTY:
RED CLOVER

Latin Name: Trifolium pratense

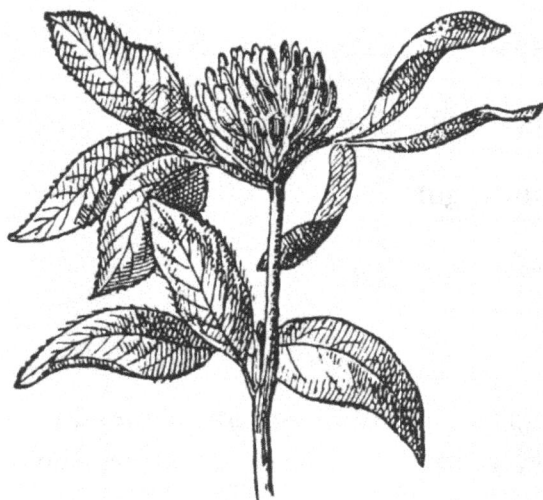

Very similar in look to the Irish 'shamrock' (trifolium repens), Red clover has both a spiritual and mythical history, with ancient Celts believing that the three leaves represented the goddess Bridget's status as maiden, mother, and crone, while St. Patrick used the shamrock to represent the Father,

Son, and Holy Ghost. The fourth leaf of rare sprigs represents faith, hope, luck, and love.

As the name "shamrock" was abandoned in parts of the western world, in favor of the name "red clover," mythology arose around that term too. Patches of clover in lawns and fields became havens for fairies, while witches were terrified of them. Even stories of Eve and Eden claim that, when she was expelled from Eden, she carried a sprig of four-leaf red clover with her. That became the basis for the legend that she carried a small bit of paradise with her.

Yet, the truth about red clover actually may be more powerful than any fable. It possesses incredible health and nutritional benefits.

Description of the Plant: red clover is a biennial or short-lived perennial with the typical clover three-leaf arrangement. It has a small (½ inch) purple or red flower head, looking something like a small bath scrubbing pompom. Flowers are very attractive to ants and bees. Several stems grow from the woody root, with the green leaves having an identifiable, conspicuously veined, white V across the leaf. Flower stems are long and thin.

Common Names: it is also known as purple clover and meadow trefoil.

How, When, and Where to Gather: red clover is a European plant that has naturalized in North America. Being a legume, it can grow in soils that are not nitrogen rich. Unfortunately, it grows well alongside corn, making it a noxious weed. Red clover does well in cool conditions, well-drained, loamy soil, wet to dry meadows, forest margins, and elevations under 8,500 feet. Its range is the eastern and central half of North America. Red clover flowers are available throughout the summer. Leaves should be picked early in the summer or throughout the spring.

Health, Nutritional, and Medicinal Benefits: alterative, antispasmodic, expectorant, sedative, phytoestrogenic, and nutritive.

Red clover is used to treat menopause symptoms, osteoporosis, asthma, whooping cough, gout, cancer, high cholesterol, bronchitis, eczema, arthritis. Red clover contains calcium, chromium, magnesium, niacin, phosphorus, potassium, thiamine, isoflavones, and Vitamin C.

Edible Parts: you can eat the flower and the leaves (early season growth).

Look-Alike Plants (Poisonous and Not): there are a few non-clover look-alikes, like vetch, and thistle which have a similar flower but a distinctly different leaf appearance. None are poisonous.

Recipe: **Red Clover Lemonade**

Ingredients

3 cups clover blossoms

6 tablespoons honey

4 cups water

1 cup lemon juice

Method:

In a saucepan, simmer clover and water for ten minutes, let cool in the refrigerator. Strain, add lemon juice and honey to the drink mix, and stir. For added flavor, sprinkle a little allspice on top of each cup.

CHAPTER TWENTY-ONE: SHEEP SORREL

Latin Name: Rumex acetosella

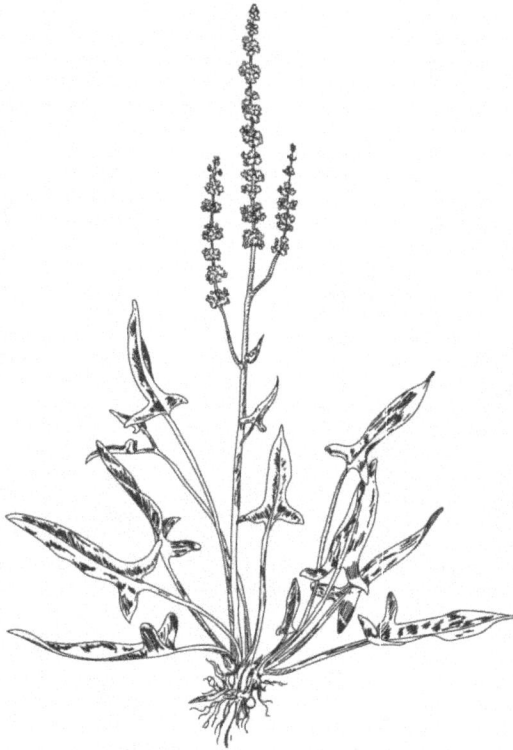

An old love potion says that, on St. Luke's Day, you should take some marigolds, thyme, a little dirt, and sheep sorrel, rub them together, then cook it over a slow fire with vinegar and honey. Then, you are to anoint yourself with this concoction before you go to bed, and chant, "St. Luke! St. Luke! Be kind to me! In my dreams let me my true love see!"

There's no certainty that this potion worked, but it certainly would have had some topical medicinal benefit.

Description of the Plant: sheep sorrel grows with a clump of long, arrow-shaped leaves arranged as a rosette from the root rhizomes under the ground. Leaves grow alternately and vary in size. Each rosette forms an upright, cone-shaped rosette of reddish flowers, each cluster on a separate stem. Male and female flowers are on separate plants, which bloom from May to October. It spreads quickly in acidic soils. Leaves have a tart, almost lemony taste.

Common Names: it is known as field sorrel and sour dock.

How, When, and Where to Gather: sheep sorrel prefers open disturbed areas, meadows and fields, pastures, utility corridors, road and rail rights-of-way, and even overgrown lawns and homesteads. It likes acidic, sandy soil or gravel, grasslands, and does not like shade. It has been naturalized to North America and now is found throughout the continent. Try to pick the leaves before late summer, as they tend to get tough, like kale. Younger leaves have a more astringent, sharp, almost lemony taste. The small seeds act as a moderate thickener for soups.

Health, Nutritional, and Medicinal Benefits: anticancer, diuretic, antioxidant, detoxifier, laxative, anti-inflammatory, diaphoretic, diuretic, refrigerant, and astringent.

Sheep sorrel, like garden sorrel, is employed as a treatment for scurvy, cancer, diarrhea, inflammation, nasal passage swelling and pain, bacterial infections, and as a diuretic.

Edible Parts: you can eat the leaves, seeds, and roots.

Look-Alike Plants (Poisonous and Not): the leaves are similar to field bindweed, which is a noxious weed but not toxic. In fact, the oxalates in sorrel can cause serious gastric distress if eaten in large quantities.

Recipe: **Creamy Sorrel Soup**

Ingredients

4 tablespoons butter

½ cup diced white onion

3 tablespoons flour

4 cups vegetable stock

6 cups chopped sorrel

¼ teaspoon salt

¼ teaspoon pepper

¼ teaspoon turmeric

2 egg yolks

½ cup cream

Method:

In a small pan, slightly caramelize the onions. In a soup pot, add the stock and bring to a simmer. Add the sorrel, onion, and spices and cook, covered, for ten minutes. Mix flour with a little cold water and add, stir, then simmer the soup for another 2-3 minutes. Let it cool in the refrigerator. Blend until smooth. In a bowl, whisk the egg yolks and cream together. Blend a bit at a time with the sorrel soup. Serve hot or cold.

CHAPTER TWENTY-TWO:
STINGING NETTLE

Latin Name: Urtica dioica

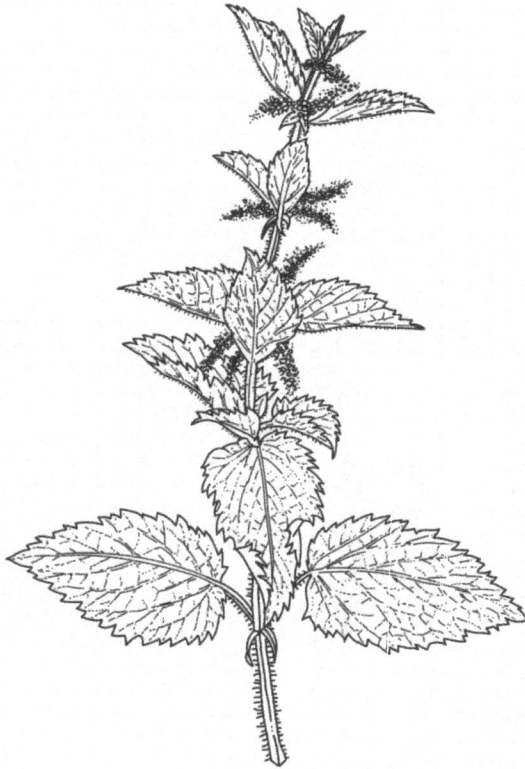

There are a few plants whose folklore and historical medicinal uses are remarkably similar to the folklore and cures of the same plant continents away, even though the two cultures never came in contact with each other. Nettle is one of them.

North American indigenous tribes told tales of the nettle as being nature's trickster, and they compared it to the coyote, devious and sly. Half a globe away, Scottish and Irish folklore referred to it as a cure for the sneaky attacks of elves, inflicting inexplicable sharp pains on them. The presence of nettle beds meant that fairies were nearby, and the nettles would catch their mischievous antics before they harmed humans. In ancient Norse mythology, Loki, the trickster god, made his fishing nets from nettles.

At the same time that North American Indians were weaving clothes from nettles to combat joint pain and arthritis, tribes in other regions and cultures in Europe and Asia were practicing urtification, or beating one's limbs with stinging nettle branches to cure aches and pains.

And, around the world, virtually everyone used nettle for the same health benefits and medicinal cures. This speaks to the strong likelihood, if not proof, that the plant has valid and effective curative properties, whether science has caught up with proving this accepted fact or not.

Description of the Plant: stinging nettle's most distinguishable feature is the fine hairs along its stems and the underside of mature leaves. Innocent-looking, they pack an incredibly irritating sting or itch. The leaves are tapered, with saw-tooth edges and divergent veins in the leaf. The plant grows to an excess of three feet in height.

Common Names: it is known as the common nettle.

How, When, and Where to Gather: while stinging nettle grows throughout the world, it is very common in most regions of North America. Nettle grows very well in damp, nitrogen-rich soils, along river and stream flood plains, old farmsteads, edges of woods including evergreen stands, and in full sun to partial shade where there is lots of humus matter and fertile soil. To avoid stings from the mature stems, harvest leaves early in the spring and summer, before they reach mature height. The mature leaves need to be cooked to avoid the stings that will be present on the hairs, mostly transferred from the stems.

Health, Nutritional, and Medicinal Benefits: anti-inflammatory, diuretic, antiseptic, mild hypoglycemic, diuretic, anti-hemorrhagic, hemostatic, detoxifier, vasodilator, circulatory stimulant, hypotensive, nutritive, galactagogue, astringent, expectorant, anti-allergic, reduces BPH, and is an anti-rheumatic.

Stinging nettle has a wide array of topical and internal medicinal uses, including treatment for gout, anemia, muscle pain, joint pain, enlarged prostate, enlarged spleen, ear and eye ailments, ulcers, and arthritis. It decreases swelling, and treats diabetes, kidney stones, and hay fever.

Edible Parts: you can eat the young leaves, stems, and roots.

Look-Alike Plants (Poisonous and Not): there are no known poisonous look-alikes for the stinging nettle.

Recipe: **Stinging Nettle Smoothie**

Ingredients

2 cups stinging nettle leaves, steamed or blanched

½ cucumber, peeled

1 cup coconut milk

1 avocado

2 bananas, overripe

1 cup lemon yogurt

1 cup pineapple

Method:

Blend all ingredients until nice and smooth, adding more yogurt as necessary for the sake of taste and consistency.

CHAPTER TWENTY-THREE:
SUMAC

Latin Name: Rhus typhina

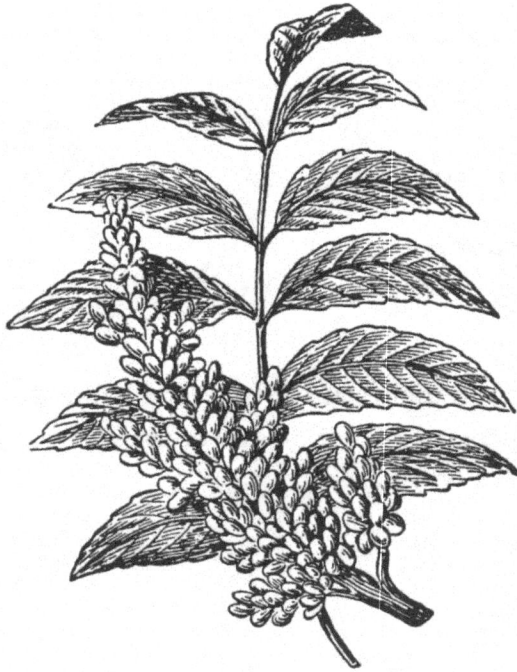

Staghorn sumac gets its name from the velvet on its stems and underside of the leaves, like the velvet on a stag's antlers in the summer.

But, native folklore also tells how the deer and elk love to conceal themselves in the fiery reddish-brown foliage of the shrub during the fall rut. The story says that the tree protects them, deceiving predators when its dry, red leaves rustle in the wind, sounding like the rustling and cracking of the stag's antlers rubbing together. The wolves, who are drawn to the sound of the leaves, are lured away from the deer, so they can carry on with their mating.

If not grounded in truth, the story still makes a wonderful children's tale.

If ever there was a need to comprehend the different varieties of plants, know the difference between sumacs. Of the trinity of poisonous plants in North America—poison ivy, poison oak, and poison sumac—sumac is the most poisonous. It looks very much like the more common staghorn sumac, except mature shrubs are smaller, and the poisonous variety grows in very wet conditions. One has the potential to kill, or make humans incredibly ill, the other is a wonderful healing and salubrious plant.

Description of the Plant: Sumac and poison sumac look similar, but, aside from habitat, there are some differences. Both have compound leaves with tapered leaflets, but the poison sumac leaf edges are smooth, while the staghorn sumac's opposite leaflet is toothed. Staghorn has nine to thirty-one leaflets, while poison sumac has, at most, unlucky thirteen. The twigs on staghorn sumac have soft hairs, while the poison sumac is smooth. Staghorn berries are round, packed tightly together in an upright tuft. Staghorn sumac grows up to twelve to twenty feet tall. The berries persist throughout the winter and leaves turn a scarlet red in the fall.

Common Names: It is known as sumac, staghorn sumac, scarlet sumac, and sumach.

How, When, and Where to Gather: Staghorn sumac and poison sumac are not the same, and grow in different habitats and terrain. Staghorn sumac grows in open areas and likes drier soils, while poison sumac prefers marshy, shaded areas. Staghorn grows on the prairies, open grasslands, old fields and abandoned yards and homesteads, roadsides, fencerows, shelterbelts, and field crop headlands. It grows south to Georgia. West to the Mississippi River valley, central plains of the Dakotas, Kansas, Utah, and the south of Manitoba, Saskatchewan, and Alberta. It grows in all Canadian provinces east of Manitoba.

Fruit is harvested in the late fall. Berries are harvested in winter, after a heavy frost, and they develop a sweet, tart taste.

Health, Nutritional, and Medicinal Benefits: it is an astringent, antiseptic, alterative, tonic, refrigerant, diuretic, emmenagogue, diaphoretic, cephalic, antidiarrheal, antioxidant, antifungal, and also anticancer.

Sumac, like mountain ash, is a mainstay food source in winter as the berries remain on the trees well into the cold season. Being very rich in antioxidants and Vitamin C, it is used to treat colds, sore throats, asthma, fever, hypoglycemia, and as an ointment or salve on open wounds.

Edible Parts: you can eat the berries (fruit).

Look-Alike Plants (Poisonous and Not): tree of heaven and poison sumac are two sumac look-alikes. Mountain ash has similar leaves and often is misidentified as sumac. Poison sumac is part of the trifecta of poisonous plants, ivy, oak, and sumac, but is, by far, the most dangerous. It grows, however, in swampy areas and is relatively uncommon.

Recipe: Staghorn Sumac Cocktails (Alcohol-Free)

Ingredients

Base:

2 cups sumac berries

4 cups water

Mix:

2 cups varied dark fruit (raspberries, strawberries, blackberries, blueberries)

3 cups tonic water or ginger ale

¼ cup orange juice

Mint or sage

Method:

Mash sumac berries in water, and let stand for four to six hours in the fridge. Remove and strain. Put varied berries in the bottom of the pitcher and mash lightly. Add sumac base and orange juice. Stir and add tonic water as the mix is still swirling. Put crushed ice in cups and pour the mixture into each cup, topping with a sprig of mint or sage.

Chapter Twenty-Four:
Sunflower

Latin Name: Helianthus spp.

It is difficult to define or describe sunflowers, simply because there are so many members of this family growing wild and domesticated. Yet, the mythology and lore surrounding these bright and cheery plants extend back to the peak of Greek civilization, and the value of sunflowers exposing themselves in unique ways.

A stranded motorist traveling in the Saskatchewan prairies a few years ago, found himself caught in a late October snowstorm. In an adjacent field was a quarter-section of sunflowers, not yet harvested. During the peak of the storm, he cut dozens of heads of sunflowers, stacked them, and built a warming fire, burning strong because of the high oil content in the seeds. It was a very practical use for a flower steeped in fairy tale mythology.

While the stranded traveler may have worshiped the sunflower during the frigid blizzard, the Greeks revered sunflowers as symbols of loyalty and adoration.

The myth is one of unrequited love. A young water nymph in love with Apollo spent endless days pining after him as he traveled across the skies, but he took no notice. Other gods did, however, rooting her into the soil where she stood, so that she could receive nourishment while she followed the sun. She became a sunflower, her yellow face always turning towards the sun.

Description of the Plant: the most identifiable part of the sunflower is its bright, face-like seed and flower head. The many varieties of sunflower also have a great diversity of sizes, from as short as eighteen inches to well over seven feet tall, with the biggest recorded at over thirty feet. The flowers, with their ring of bright tapered petals and center reproductive florets, may be yellow, white, red, orange, or purple. The heads may be as small as a few inches in diameter, or over a foot across. There may be over 1,000 florets, which each produces a single seed. The stems are hollow (pithy), woody, and round with vertical ridges. Leaves are pinnated, oblong, and pointed at the end. Flowers bloom from mid-summer to early autumn, with the outer petals remaining while the floret produces its seed and the seed matures. Unless consumed by birds, bears, raccoons, or skunks, the seed heads will remain well into the winter.

Common Names: it is also known as a giant aster.

How, When, and Where to Gather: sunflower varieties grow domestically and wild throughout almost all of North America, including southern Alaska, Yukon, and Northwest Territories. It likes prairies, grasslands, dry, sunny, and open areas, edges of cropland, and old homestead yards. It can grow well in moist, disturbed soils. Many domestic varieties now grow wild and are known as "volunteer" sunflowers. Seed heads can be harvested in early autumn, after they have ripened and dried. Roots may be harvested from late summer through early winter, while leaves are best harvested in early to late spring. Stems may be consumed at any time, but are best in early to mid-summer. Flowers may be picked in early to mid-summer.

Health, Nutritional, and Medicinal Benefits: antioxidant, antimicrobial, anti-inflammatory, antihypertensive, wound-healing, cardiovascular, diuretic, and expectorant.

The sunflower, like the cattail, is exceptionally versatile. Both are used for heat, with the sunflower seeds providing oil and thick stalks for fuel. Both are rich in nutrients and healthy starches. Sunflower infusions were used for chest pains and pulmonary issues. The seeds were sometimes used as a stimulant,providing energy to voyagers on long treks. It is used to treat fevers, coughs, and colds, to cauterize wounds, and as a kidney or bladder cleanse.

*Edible Part*s: you can eat the root, young leaves, seeds, flower petals, and stems.

Look-Alike Plants (Poisonous and Not): there are many sunflower varieties and, consequently, many look-alikes, but none are toxic.

Recipe: **Grilled Sunflower Heads**

Ingredients

1 large immature sunflower head (seeds not hardened and ripe)

3-4 slices bacon, cooked and crumbled, bacon fat retained

¼ cup avocado oil

¼ onion, diced fine

1 tablespoon red chili flakes

2 cloves garlic, chopped fine

salt to taste

Method:

Mix together bacon fat and oil. In a large roasting pan, set sunflower head, sprinkle bacon pieces, onion, and garlic over the head. Top with chili flakes and salt. Spray oil over the head generously. Barbeque covered for twenty minutes, then remove, and spritz with lemon juice.

CHAPTER TWENTY-FIVE:
THISTLE

Latin Name: Silybum marianum (milk thistle), Cirsium arvense (canada thistle)

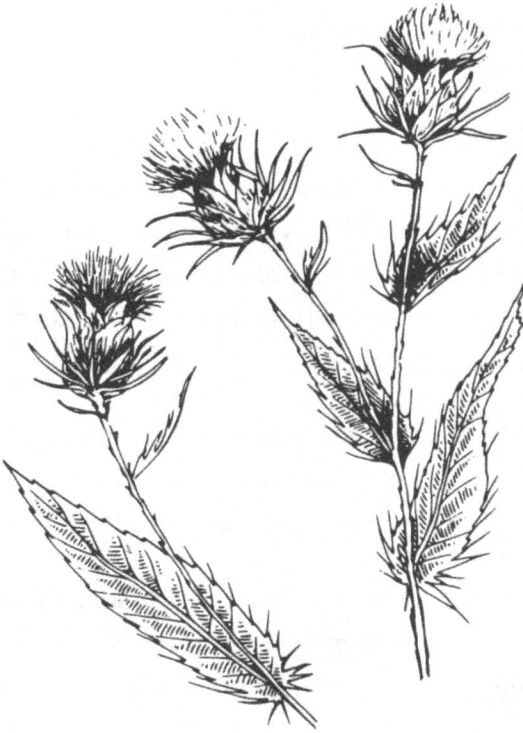

This flower finds itself at the center of numerous mythological tales and the folklore of many countries. In Scotland, it signifies devotion and bravery. In the Basque region of France, it is the herb of witches. A garland of thistle or a bunch hung over a doorway protects against their evil influence. Before the crown of brambles that Christ wore, a crown or cape of thistles was seen as punishment, but also of healing and strength.

There are more than 200 species of thistle worldwide, 58 in North America alone. The most commonly grown type for medicinal use would be the milk thistle, closely followed by the sow thistle (a member of the aster family, similar in appearance to the dandelion) and the Canada (creeping) thistle.

All thistles have been common staples in early North American indigenous diets. As some species from Europe found their way into the wilds of Canada and the United States, indigenous folks embraced them for their medicinal properties, as they did with scores of other plants that found their way across the ocean.

The national flower of Scotland, the spear thistle, is now more common in North America than in Scotland, but it has been present in the New World for less than 350 years.

Description of the Plant: milk thistle's identifying marks are the white veins on its prickly, bright green leaves. Flower heads are bright purple with spiny bracts around the flower base. Leaves and stems all have stiff spines. Sow thistle is a tall plant (three feet), with few branching stems except near the top where the flowers occur. Blooms look like smaller dandelion flowers. The leaves are alternate, odd pinnate, becoming smaller as they approach the top. Their prickles are soft. Canada thistle has prickly stems and stalkless leaves. Flowers are smaller than other thistles. There are no spines on the many bracts at the base of the flowers. It grows up to four feet tall. Russian thistle is otherwise known as tumbleweed.

Common Names: it is known as milk thistle, sow thistle, Canada thistle, creeping thistle, California thistle, and field thistle.

How, When, and Where to Gather: the many varieties of thistle in North America mean that thistle grows in a variety of locations and soil conditions. They will grow in moist to dry spots, urban and rural areas, disturbed sites such as wastelands, old homesteads and yards, roadsides, ditches and utility rights-of-way, trails, logging roads, vacant land, pastures, and cultivated farmland. They generally are designated as noxious weeds. Thistle from Europe has naturalized across all of North America, along with native species. They prefer sunny, open areas and thrive around manure piles.

Harvesting periods of the thistle depend upon the part of the thistle you are foraging. Roots may be harvested throughout the growing season and well into winter. However, as the season progresses and if the plant is growing in gravelly, dry conditions, the roots will be smaller, tougher, and more bark-like. Older plants (older than two years) will have larger roots, while this year's growth will have small, more tender roots. The seed pod or heads can be harvested in mid to late summer, a week or so after the flower has bloomed and before the "parachutes" on the seed develop and the seed pod breaks open. The leaves are best picked no later than early summer, as they tend to develop larger prickles and become more veiny and tough. They develop a bitter taste as the summer progresses.

Health, Nutritional, and Medicinal Benefits: anti-diabetic, anti-cancer, and antioxidant.

Milk thistle is used as liver treatment for cirrhosis, jaundice, and hepatitis, to lower cholesterol, manage Type 2 diabetes, and treat gallbladder disorders. Thistle has antioxidant properties and is used to treat heart disease.

Edible Parts: you can eat the root (peeled), stems (peeled), seed head (medicinal), and flower base (and flower, in some varieties).

Look-Alike Plants (Poisonous and Not): many thistles look similar, but some have softer spines on their leaves than others. Even dandelions have a similar leaf to a sow thistle. Hemlock has a similar growth pattern and looks somewhat alike, but has more fern-like leaves. You should know it is also deadly poisonous!

Recipe: **Thistle in Almond Sauce**

Ingredients

2 cups thistle leaves, cleaned with hard veining removed

1.5 teaspoons garlic powder

⅓ teaspoon pepper

salt to taste

3 tablespoons almond flakes or crumbled walnuts

1 cup almond flour

½ cup parmesan cheese

Method:

Cook thistles in two cups of water until tender. Drain, and cool the liquid. Add in garlic powder, pepper, and salt, stirring. Blend in almond flour until no lumps appear. Simmer for several minutes, stirring often to avoid scorching. Once it thickens, pour over thistle, then stir in parmesan and top with almond flakes. You may spritz with a little lemon for more zest and tang.

CHAPTER TWENTY-SIX:
VIOLET

Latin Name: Viola odorata

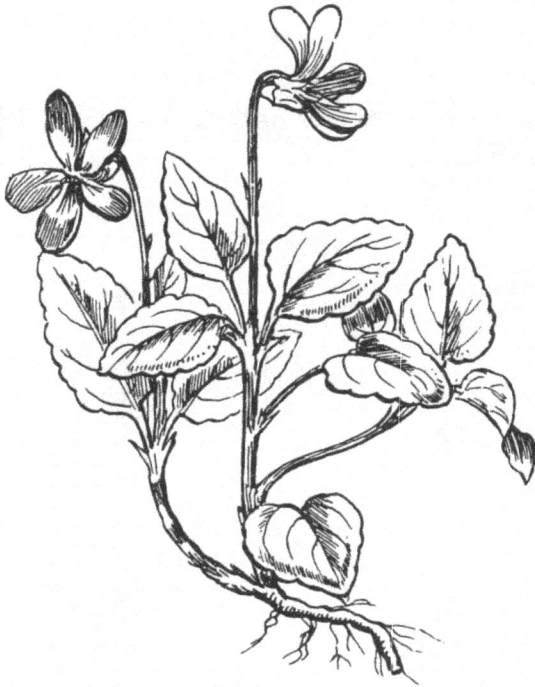

Did you know the Greeks and Romans associated violets with death and funerals? They scattered them around tombs, and as a symbol of innocence, they blanketed children's graves with the flowers. The hope was that the children would rise quickly to the heavens.

The common moniker for the violet—johnny-jump-up—arose from how quickly this little bloom sprouts in the spring, almost appearing to jump out of the soil. Wild violets do emerge quickly and propagate abundantly in open meadows, but they do not invade spaces in the way that many weeds do.

Description of the Plant: there are over 600 species of violet, none are toxic. They have heart-shaped, scalloped leaves, but a few are alternate linear or palmate. They are mostly smaller plants. Flowers have five petals, two swept upward, two to the sides, and one broad petal downward. Seed pods look somewhat like small pea pods, with five per flower head.

Common Names: viola, Johnny-jump-up.

How, When, and Where to Gather: violets are native to most areas of North America, primarily in central and eastern Canada and the United States. They are found in Europe, but are not as common as in North America. There are many species of violets, all non-toxic and mostly edible. They prefer shady, moist, fertile soil but often are found at the edges of lawns (johnny jump-ups and violas). The flowers appear delicate but are very hardy and even cold-tolerant. They grow in many environments, including woodlands, dry desert conditions, and marshy areas. Violet flowers produce well in early spring to mid-summer. Leaves remain relatively tender and flavorful throughout the growing season. Seeds, although edible, are very small and difficult to gather.

Health, Nutritional, and Medicinal Benefits: it is an anti-inflammatory, antimicrobial, demulcent, expectorant, lymphagogue, vulnerary, antitumor, antirheumatic, diuretic, and also used as a laxative.

Violet flowers often accompany lavender and chamomile in sachets to be placed under pillows and induce sleep. It is a sleep aid when used as tea. The petals ease inflammation externally, soothing skin irritations, sores, puffy eyes, and even hemorrhoids. Violet also is good for the lymphatic system.

Edible Parts: you can eat the leaves, flowers, and seeds.

Look-Alike Plants (Poisonous and Not): lesser celandine has similar leaves to violet and is poisonous, but it has yellow flowers that look nothing like the blooms of the violet plant.

Recipe: Violet Ice

Ingredients

2 cups violet flowers plus 1 cup violet flowers

3 cups water

3 tablespoons cane sugar

juice from 1 lemon

Method:

Simmer two cups of violet flowers and sugar in water for five to seven minutes. Remove and let cool. Stir in lemon juice. Pour mixture into ice cube trays, then add one or two violet flowers to each cube. Freeze. Serve with fruit fizzy cocktails.

CHAPTER TWENTY-SEVEN:
WILD GARLIC

Latin name: Allium ursinum

Dracula and vampires were merely literary extensions of the belief that garlic could ward off the evil spirits and influences that the medieval world believed caused illness. This recognition of the power of garlic extends worldwide, wherever garlic grows.

Garlic is either a lifesaver or protector against demons (according to lore), a stinky and useless root or an amazing pantry of health benefits (according to the consumers' personal bias). Regardless, people have relied on it for use in thousands of recipes for flavor and scores of medicinal and health benefits, for nearly five thousand years of documented history.

Its power to ward off illness exceeds that of the apple, in the old saying, "an apple a day keeps the doctor away." The Welsh slogan, "Eat leeks in March and garlic in May. Then the rest of the year, your doctor can play," sums up belief in its preventative power over disease.

Description of the Plant: wild garlic leaf is shaped like a long willow leaf, narrow at the base, flying slightly, and tapered to a point at the apex. It is a bright green color. They grow from the base of the plant, with several growing randomly out. The flowers are small and white, star-shaped, several growing from numerous stalks at the top of a stem. The garlic is easily identified by its pungent smell.

Common Names: it is also called wild cow leek and bear garlic.

How, When, and Where to Gather: wild garlic is native to North America, with varieties growing across the entire continent. They like shady areas, deciduous forests, moist soils, slightly acidic soils , and lowlands. They are found occasionally in scrubland and hedgerows or field headlands bordering waterways. In addition to the numerous varieties of wild garlic, there are several species of wild onion that look very similar, as well as chives that have naturalized in the wild. Cultivated garlic, introduced by European settlers, has now naturalized and grows wild. It is often found alongside horseradish and hawthorn in old farmyards and abandoned homesteads.

Health, Nutritional, and Medicinal Benefits: it is antibacterial, antifungal, immunomodulator, antispasmodic, carminative, antithrombotic, cardioprotective, antimicrobial, diaphoretic, expectorant, hepatoprotective, hypoglycemic, hypolipidemic, hypotensive, and rubefacient.

Wild garlic, like most wild plants, provides all the benefits of the cultivated version, but it is more potent. It helps to lower blood pressure, reduces cholesterol, reduces inflammation, decreases insulin sensitivity, inhibits platelet aggregation, and eases stomach pain. It treats asthma and bronchitis, aids in weight loss, treats intestinal ailments, and relieves indigestion. Externally, it can be applied to arthritic joints. Garlic, with plantain, aids in relieving the itch of poison ivy and can help heal sores.

Edible Parts: you can eat the stem, root, and flowers.

Look-Alike Plants (Poisonous and Not): lily of the valley, with its attractive, small, white, bell-shaped flowers is quite poisonous, and looks something like wild garlic. "Star of Jerusalem" flowers grow in the same conditions as wild garlic. are similar in look, and non-edible, though not poisonous.

Recipe: **Wild Garlic Paste**

Ingredients

½ pound wild garlic leaves

½ ounce sea salt

½ cup coconut oil, softened

Method:

Blend all ingredients in a blender, pour into a container, and let set. Coconut oil solidifies at room temperature. You may store the paste for up to a month in the refrigerator.

Chapter Twenty-Eight:
Wild Ginger

Latin Name: Asarum canadense

Folklore holds that eating ginger before magic rituals increases the power of that magic. It is used in love spells, to attract money and power, and to ensure success in personal and business endeavors.

The wild ginger found in North America is quite different from that found in Europe and even more so from cultivated ginger. North American wild ginger sometimes is known as snakeroot, partly because of the winding nature of its rhizomes that knot together to look like intertwined snakes, and partly because it was used to treat snake bites.

This practice of using plants that resembled the ailment or part of the body that they were used to treat was a common thread in First Nations folklore. Oddly, it has been borne out often in various medicinal cures they used.

Settlers introduced their own mythologies into the harvesting of wild ginger, believing that they should use only cold steel (not tempered), to harvest. This may have been intended to preserve its sharp, sweet, and spicy flavor, more than for mythological reasons.

During the Roman holiday, Saturnalia, people hung the bitter herbs (wild ginger, olive, bindwood, holly, horsetail) in their homes as a tribute to the god Saturn.

Description of the Plant: wild ginger leaves are heart-shaped, growing on a slender, long (two to three inch) stem that looks similar to nasturtium stems. The stems grow out of the knotty root that looks like numerous small snakes intertwined. Leaves are palmated, somewhat like coltsfoot leaves. They have an almost furry appearance underneath.

Common Names: wild ginger, Canada ginger.

How, When, and Where to Gather: ginger grows in the thicker undergrowth of woods, moist low-elevation forests of the Pacific Northwest, in British Columbia, Oregon, Washington, California, Idaho, Montana, and western Alberta. Some have been found in Minnesota and southern Ontario. It prefers mild, wet winters and warm, dry summers. It also grows in eastern North America in spotty growth regions.

Health, Nutritional, and Medicinal Benefits: it is useful as an anti-inflammatory, stimulant, anti-colic, anti-anxiety, anti-stress, antiseptic, antibacterial, and anti-asthmatic.

Wild ginger's most popular use is to relieve upset stomachs, indigestion, and intestinal ailments, such as gas and cramps. It is also used to treat arthritis, colds, fibromyalgia, influenza, lupus, and high cholesterol.

Edible Parts: you can eat the root and the stem (in moderation).

Look-Alike Plants (Poisonous and Not): wild ginger often is cross-identified with coltsfoot, or local viola species. Ginger flowers grow at the base of the plant near the ground. The coltsfoot leaf, though, is not heart-shaped like the wild ginger plant.

Recipe: **Wild Ginger Chocolate Treats**

Ingredients

½ pound wild ginger roots, broken into segments

1 package mint or semi-sweet chocolate chips

Method:

Melt chocolate chips in a double boiler. Stir in ginger root. Remove them from the chocolate, and place the roots spaced out on a sheet of wax paper to cool and solidify.

CHAPTER TWENTY-NINE:
WILD GRAPE

Latin Name: Vitis riparia

Why did the Viking explorers, when landing in the new world, name it "Vinland?" The smell of the grapes was so overpowering that they believed the entire land must be covered by them. This may be a bit of a yarn, since they also, quite sarcastically, called an island of nothing but glaciers and ice in the coldest part of their world, Greenland!

Grapes have a long history of being loved (as fruit and wine), around the world with the ancient Greeks having a god, Dionysus, dedicated to wine and grapes. According to legend, he pursued Ampelos recklessly, who was gored to death by a bull. Dionysus changed his dead lover into a grapevine. Perhaps it is a confusing and twisted legend, but it is consistent with the twisting nature of the grapevine itself.

Description of the Plant: wild grapes always have heart-shaped leaves, although the leaves mostly have toothed margins and a simple alternate pattern. In some cases, they are shaped somewhat like a poplar leaf with jagged edges, but larger and have a heart indentation at the stem. There may be three or five lobes on the leaves. The plants have forked tendrils that dry out as they age. Plants last for years, and many stems do not die back in winter, becoming more brittle and gnarled as they age. Flowers look shaggy, form in a droopy cluster, and develop into bunches of grapes.

Common Names: they are also known as fox grapes.

How, When, and Where to Gather: wild grapes originally grew on the east coast Appalachian area and the west coast of North America, including Oregon and California. It has spread to other coastal ranges, the central valley, and Sierra foothills. It prefers creeks, streams, and floodplains below 3,200 feet in elevation. California grape grows in the Sierra foothills.

Health, Nutritional, and Medicinal Benefits: it is an analgesic, anti-inflammatory, cardiotonic, disinfectant, antioxidant, and antidiarrheal.

Grape leaf tea is used to treat diarrhea, stomach ache, hepatitis, and thrush. Grape leaf poultice, applied externally, treats headache, rheumatism, fevers, coughs, and sore throat. Grape root, as a wash, is used to treat sore eyes. The fruit is beneficial in preventing cardiovascular disease, reducing bad cholesterol, and protecting against cancer. The grapeseed oil also helps with cholesterol levels and heart health. Seeds and fruit are indicated in helping to improve motor skills and memory and to fight cell aging, thanks to resveratrol. The leaves also help blood circulation.

Edible Parts: you can eat the fruit, leaf, and root.

Look-Alike Plants (Poisonous and Not): common moonseed and porcelain berry both look similar to wild grapes and both are poisonous.

Recipe: **Fermented Grape Leaves**

Ingredients

4-6 cups grape leaves

¼ cup pickling salt

4 cups filtered water

Method:

Roll grape leaves tightly in bundles about the size of a fist. Stuff them in quart-sized mason jars. Mix salt and water. Pour over grape leaves and cover loosely. Let ferment for three weeks until the process stops, then seal and store. Ideal for stuffed grape leaf recipes.

CHAPTER THIRTY:
WILD MINT

Latin Name: Mentha arvensis, Mentha canadensis

The scent of mint is prominent in mythology. Its smell is so powerful that it historically has been used to mask the smell of carrion and the decay of corpses. This led mint naturally into myths involving Hades, the god of death and the underworld, Persephone, the queen of the underworld, and Menthe, a nymph with whom Hades was enamored. In typical tragic fashion, Persephone jealously turned Menthe to dust, from which Hades grew mint.

There are so many members of the mint family growing wild that it is difficult to establish a dominant set of myths or lore associated with them. From catnip to lemon balm, peppermint to spearmint, they have captured the taste buds of the world.

Description of the Plant: Mints have very fragrant, toothed leaves and tiny purple to white flowers. In most species, the margins look almost like the teeth of a circular saw, in others, the toothed edges are smoother. They grow between eighteen inches and four feet high, depending on variety, on angled, square, green, hairy stems. The mints have whorls of flowers that bloom in early summer.

Common Names: it is known as catnip, catmint, peppermint, spearmint, bee mint, lemon mint, and lemon balm.

How, When, and Where to Gather: wild mint grows across all of North America. There are many members of the mint family. It likes growing around moist meadows, wetlands, and marshes, full to part sun, softer soils, and nitrogen-rich growing mediums. Some varieties, such as the balms, grow well in sun, while spearmint tolerates shade well.

Health, Nutritional, and Medicinal Benefits: it is an anticatarrhal, tonic, diaphoretic, anthelmintic, bitter, digestive, choleretic, emmenagogue, and diuretic.

The multitude of mint family members means there is a multitude of medicinal, culinary, and health uses for this plant.

Mint has been recognized for centuries as a digestive aid, calmative for upset stomachs, breath freshener, stress, and anxiety reducer, and sleep aid. Peppermint is well known for its calming effect on the digestive system, while lemon or bee balm is an effective mosquito repellent. Catnip, or catmint, protects against harmful bacteria, while spearmint is a popular mouthwash or toothpaste additive. High in antioxidants, mints are excellent anti-aging, cancer-inhibiting herbs. They maintain healthy skin and assist with allergy relief. Mints are used to treat cold symptoms, promote urine flow, relieve thirst, strengthen kidney function, treat asthma, liver and spleen disorders, relieve sore throat, cough, inflammation, and aching joints, and alleviate muscle spasms.

Edible Parts: you can eat the leaves and the flowers.

Look-Alike Plants (Poisonous and Not): bugleweed and northern horehound both look like mints, but are relatively safe and non-toxic, like almost all members of the mint family.

***Recipe*: Mint Peas**

Ingredients

4 cups shelled peas or edible pod peas

½ medium red onion, thinly sliced

½ cup mint leaves, torn small

vinaigrette

Method:

In a bowl mix all ingredients and let stand for 60 minutes, stirring occasionally.

CHAPTER THIRTY-ONE:
WILD ONION

Latin Name: Allium canadense

While many herbs and medicinal plants also have myths and folklore associated with them, the onion's history is rooted in practical applications. It was such a valued food that the Jews, when leaving Egypt, lamented the loss of the onion in their diet. The southwest indigenous people of North America hold annual festivals in honor of the onion. Recently, a 1,300-year-old onion was discovered in a woman's grave.

Like garlic, they have been used to ward off evil and keep witches or spirits away. They are revered, not as something mysterious, but as an essential part of a healthy diet, and have been for thousands of years. As a result of their perceived value, modern cultivated onions began as the small, shallot-style wild onion, bred and nurtured until the modern yellow, white, Spanish, red, and other varieties became perfected.

Description of the Plant: it is a monocot, with many singular stems/leaves erupting from the base. The stems are wedgy, triangular in cross-section, and hollow, producing a white flower at the end of most of the stems. Chives, onions, and garlic produce purple flowers, sometimes white. The stems resemble garlic and chives more than domestic onion.

Common Names: it is known as meadow onion or Canada garlic.

How, When, and Where to Gather: wild onion grows in full to partial sun, mid-range soil moisture, and slightly acidic soils. It grows well in meadows, grassy wooded banks of creeks, and in marshy areas. It can be found along roadsides and railroad embankments, spread by human traffic. It predominates in eastern North America, but there are varieties throughout the continent, often where wild garlic is found. Gather it in spring, summer, and autumn. The stems are best before they begin to dry and droop in the summer heat, but, as a perennial, they regrow each year, so it is possible actually to harvest the root well into winter, before the frost is deep and the cold collapses the root bulb.

Health, Nutritional, and Medicinal Benefits: it is an anti-inflammatory, antibacterial, antifungal, immunomodulator, antispasmodic, carminative, antithrombotic, cardioprotective, antimicrobial, diaphoretic, expectorant, hepatoprotective, hypoglycemic, hypolipidemic, hypotensive, and rubefacient.

Wild onion, like wild garlic, has an array of medicinal and health benefits. It is pain-relieving and helps treat inflammation, muscle aches, and sprains. It is cardio-tonic, strengthening the heart muscle, while also stabilizing irregular heartbeats. Onion is used to treat skin infections, rashes, boils, and warts. It is used to remove intestinal worms and helps relieve gas and bloating.

Edible Parts: you can eat the root, stem, leaf, blossom, and the seed bulb.

Look-Alike Plants (Poisonous and Not): death camas and crow poison both are poisonous plants that look like wild onions. Chives, which now grow wild, also look like wild onion, but are very safe to eat.

Recipe: Wild Onion Scrambled Eggs

Ingredients

½ cup chopped wild onion

5 eggs

½ teaspoon turmeric

salt to taste

½ teaspoon garlic powder

¼ teaspoon red chili flakes

1 tablespoon butter, melted

cooking oil

Method:

Scramble eggs in a bowl, sprinkling in turmeric, garlic powder, and butter. In a warm fry pan with oil, add in onions and chile and cook until softened. Add in your eggs, moving the curds around as they cook. Turn off the heat and gently guide them into doneness. Do not overcook!

CHAPTER THIRTY-TWO:
WILD ROSE

Latin Name: Rosa rugosa, Rosa canina, Rosa multiflora, and more

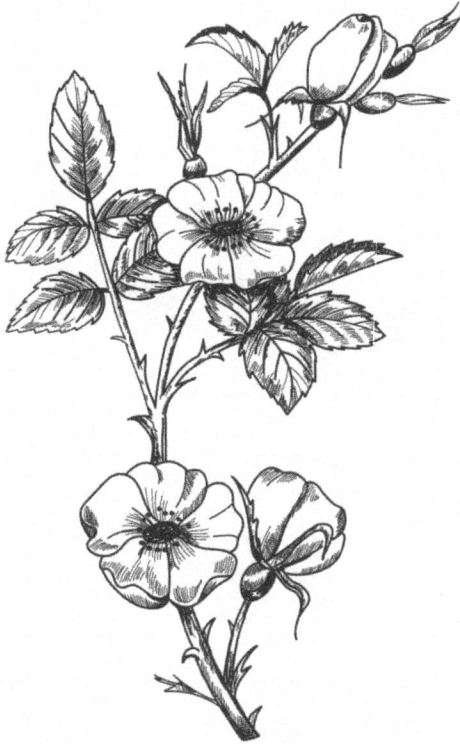

The mythology surrounding the rose is a confusing one, with early Christians believing it was the blood of Christ that stained the white rose red. In Roman mythology, the goddess of flowers, Flora, created the rose from the body of a nymph.

In Greek mythology, Aphrodite, while pursuing Adonis, cut her feet on thorns, drawing blood that became roses. The wild roses of North America also held religious symbolism for the Indigenous peoples. They believed roses to be the symbol of life, keeping ghosts away.

Description of the Plant: wild rose offers the figurative carrot and stick approach: the beautiful, delicate flowers contrast with the very sharp thorns the plant uses as a defense. Flowers are bright pink to almost white, depending on the quality and type of soil in which they grow and the flower always has five petals. Compound leaves grow with seven to nine dark green shiny leaflets that are oval with sharp, saw-tooth edges. The shrubs grow to about three feet, but tend to bend over as they grow larger. The flowers ripen into reddish-orange fruits, called hips. *Common Names*: it is also known as sweet briar or dog rose.

How, When, and Where to Gather: wild roses are found from Alaska to Atlantic Canada. It endures cold winters, and grows in open areas, prairie fields, clearings, roadsides, trails, and other open areas. It also likes thickets and small stands of brush, stream banks, and rocky outcrops. Pick the flowers in mid-summer to late summer, and the rosehips (seed pods) in late summer through to early winter. Leaves should be picked in limited quantities only until early to mid-summer, as the dry season will stress the plants.

Health, Nutritional, and Medicinal Benefits: it is a diuretic, digestive, mildly sedative, antiseptic, anti-inflammatory, anti-parasitic, laxative, anti-cholesterol, antispasmodic, and emmenagogue.

Rose hips and rose petal teas, emulsions, tinctures, and decoctions reduce pain. Rose is used as a heart tonic, to lower cholesterol, treat gout, for sore throats, to stimulate the liver, and increase appetite and circulation. Rose petals are mild laxatives, work as antispasmodic, relieve intestinal cramping, help soothe the nervous system, and ease tension. Topically, rose can treat inflammation in wounds, rashes, bites, stings, and hives. Rose hips have excellent nutritional value, with many vitamins, minerals, and iron.

Edible Parts: you can eat the flower, rose hip, and leaves (tea).

Look-Alike Plants (Poisonous and Not): there are no toxic look-alikes for the wild rose.

Recipe: **Wild Rose Oatmeal**

Ingredients

1 cup steel cut oatmeal

2 cups rose petals

½ cup blanched rose hips

½ cup raisins or dried cranberries

½ cup chopped apples

¼ teaspoon cinnamon

Method:

Make oatmeal according to instructions, with rose hips, cranberries, and apples. Add in cinnamon. Serve in bowls and top with rose petals and a light sprinkling of cane sugar.

CHAPTER THIRTY-THREE:
WILD SARSAPARILLA

Latin Name: Aralia nudicaulis

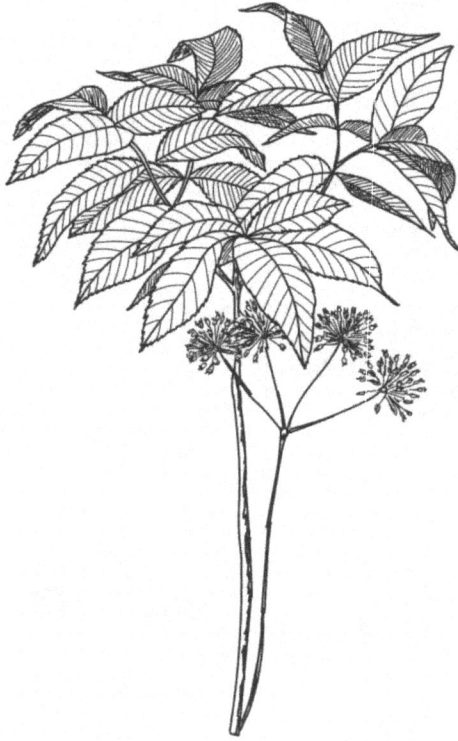

In the Greek myths of Krokos and Smilax, Smilax pursues Krokos, but he is not interested. She wastes away, and Aphrodite turns her into a briar that smells like carrion and has berries as black as night—the sarsaparilla vine.

Aficionados of old Western movies may be forgiven for thinking that the sarsaparilla drink that the pure, dressed-in-white hero cowboy drank actually was made from the root of the sarsaparilla plant. Alas, it was not. Most often, it was made from birch oil.

Yet, sarsaparilla commonly grows as a trailing vine in the southwest United States, South America, tropical Central America, and the west coast rain forests of British Columbia. It often is confused with yellow dock, but yellow dock is actually related to several varieties of sorrel.

Description of the Plant: once this plant was uncommon in northern temperate climates, but now it is found even in Manitoba. It has a strong resemblance to poison ivy and likes similar conditions, so care must be exercised when selecting the plant. Sarsaparilla has a single leaf stalk that divides into three stems, each with three to five oval to pointed, toothless, oblong-shaped leaflets. Flowers are greenish white, on three umbels on a separate flowering stem.

Common Names: it is also known as wild licorice.

How, When, and Where to Gather: sarsaparilla grows in full shade and semi-shaded areas. Its range includes Alberta to Newfoundland, south as far as Georgia, in Nebraska, and North Dakota, but it is less common in the prairie regions. There is some growth in the northwestern United States and British Columbia. Sarsaparilla is relatively adaptable to varied site requirements. It grows in coarse, fine, and medium textured soil, ground that is moderate to rich in nutrients, and poorly drained to well-drained sites. It is shade-tolerant, but it prefers lightly shaded, open woods.

Health, Nutritional, and Medicinal Benefits: it is a pituitary stimulant, metabolic stimulant, immuno-stimulant, antiseptic, antibiotic, alterative, anti-inflammatory, antipruritic, anti-rheumatic, diaphoretic, alterative, aphrodisiac, testosteronic, progesteronic, diuretic, and vulnerary.

Externally, sarsaparilla is used as a poultice for wounds, burns, sore muscles, joint pain, insect bites, eczema, or sores. The root, in a tincture or decoction, is used as a cough medicine, to treat asthma, pulmonary diseases, rheumatism, digestive issues, stomach aches, and toothaches.

Edible Parts: you can eat the root, leaves, and fruit (in limited quantities).

Look-Alike Plants (Poisonous and Not): poison ivy and sarsaparilla look similar early in the spring, but not as they mature.

Recipe: **Sarsaparilla Root Beer**

Ingredients

1 cup chopped sarsaparilla root

4 cups water

½ teaspoon anise

½ teaspoon allspice

1 stick cinnamon

¼ cup molasses

1 cup demerara sugar

8 cups soda water

Method:

To the water add all spices and root, simmer for thirty minutes. Add molasses and simmer for another five minutes. Remove from heat and filter. Add liquid back to pot, bring to a simmer and add sugar. Remove from heat and cool. Pour into glasses about ⅓ full, add ice, and then fill with soda water.

CHAPTER THIRTY-FOUR:
WILD STRAWBERRY

Latin Name: Fragaria vesca, Fragaria alpina

One only has to look at the shape of the strawberry to understand its symbolism in lore and mythology: heart-shaped. It also has a similar shape to an enlarged womb. So, as expected, it is both symbolic of love and of fertility. Strawberry was used as a marker around the entrances, altars, and pillars of early Christian churches. For the Romans, it also represented the goddess of love—Venus.

In contrast, Anne Boleyn's strawberry-shaped red birthmark indicated that she actually was a witch! England broke with the Roman Catholic church following the annulment of Henry VIII's marriage to his first wife. Henry VIII then took a second wife—Anne Boleyn. Her haughty attitude, the "evil" wife who followed Queen Catherine, and her inability to bear a son for the king all led to the court disliking her and seeking reasons to condemn her. If she was a witch, it did not save her from being beheaded on May 19, 1536. Her strawberry birthmark also did not save her.

Description of the Plant: wild strawberries look identical to cultivated ones, except that they are widespread throughout fields and much smaller. The fruit is more diminutive, the plant leaves are not as large, and the entire plant is not as robust. However, the berries are as nutritious or more so than domestic ones, and the leaves have more nutrients.

Leaves are pinnate and have three leaflets with toothed edges and a somewhat hairy surface. Flowers are small and white, with five rounded petals.

Common Names: it is known as the alpine strawberry.

How, When, and Where to Gather: wild strawberry, or alpine strawberry, is a very flexible, adaptable fruit, with a wide range of habitats. These include mixed woods and hardwood forests, edges of cedar and evergreen swamps and moss, rocky woodlands, and damp ledges. It also thrives in rich, loamy drier soil, and will grow even in gravelly areas and wasteland, in yards, and along trails and pathways. Spread by birds, bears, and even humans, their seeds grow wherever there are enough nutrients to germinate. They are found throughout the United States and Canada, as far north as central Alaska. Fruit is ready to be picked in late June to early July in northern parts of North America, and a few weeks earlier in the south. Leaves may be picked throughout the growing season. However, in later summer, bugs tend to scar the leaves and lay eggs on the undersides.

Health, Nutritional, and Medicinal Benefits: it is a laxative, diuretic, astringent, depurative, antirheumatic, anti-inflammatory, and antioxidant.

Strawberries have an extensive history in folklore as a medicinal herb. Leaves and flowers were used to treat gout but are not as widely used as in the past. However, they are still beneficial for people suffering from dysentery, gout, arthritis, premature aging, high blood pressure, high cholesterol, diabetes, liver damage, a weak immune system, high toxicity, cancer risks, sore throat, to promote eye health, cardiovascular system, respiratory infections, indigestion, constipation, dehydration, and to improve kidney function.

Edible Parts: you can eat the leaves and the seeds (fruit).

Look-Alike Plants (Poisonous and Not): the closest look-alike to a wild strawberry is strawberry weed, which does not produce the distinctive berries and is not toxic.

Recipe: Strawberry Liqueur

Ingredients

2 cups strawberries, chopped

1 ½ cup white sugar

2 cups vodka

Method:

Place strawberries in a mason jar. Mix vodka and sugar and pour over strawberries. Let sit for six weeks, shaking occasionally. Filter liquid into jars and store in the refrigerator.

CHAPTER THIRTY-FIVE:
WOOD SORREL

Latin Name: Oxalis acetosella

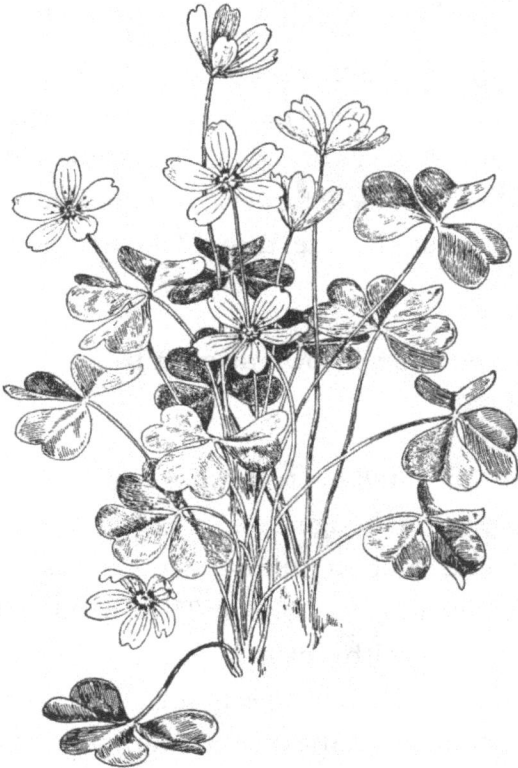

A large number of medicinal plants also carry religious symbolism. Wood sorrel is one such plant. The veins of the leaves are said to represent the marks of the blood of Christ. Part of its connection to Christian mythology arises from its tendency to flower between the Easter holiday and Whitsun, coinciding with the rising of Christ. It also blooms a second time in the UK in late summer to early fall.

It also has been associated with the Irish shamrock. Although it is related to garden and field sorrel, it looks completely dissimilar but has a similar, lemony taste. Garden and field sorrel look more like a swiss chard leaf without the long stem.

Description of the Plant: wood sorrel leaves look similar to clover leaves, with three heart-shaped segments. Leaves grow in clusters. Flowers are small and white with five petals. They produce two crops of flowers, but generally only the first germinates. The stems are thin, delicate, and tasty, often turning reddish.

Common Names: it is known as sour trefoil, sour grass, and yellow oxalis.

How, When, and Where to Gather: as the name implies, wood sorrel prefers hedgerows, shaded areas, areas with filtered light like that in thinner woodlands, and in creek banks, and other moist habitats. They need rich, moist soil like that provided with rotting leaf cover, and need good drainage to thrive. Their range is all of North America from southern Canada to Tennessee in the southeast, westward to Minnesota, and south along the Dakotas. Wood sorrel leaves and flowers are best in spring and early summer.

Health, Nutritional, and Medicinal Benefits: it is used as a diuretic, astringent, anticancer, and anti-nausea.

Applied to the skin, wood sorrel provides a soothing effect. It is used to treat scurvy, urinary tract infections, fever, sore throats, mouth sores, nausea, cleanse the blood, and act as an anticancer treatment.

Edible Parts: you can eat the leaves, flowers, and stems.

Look-Alike Plants (Poisonous and Not): wood sorrel looks like clovers and black medic, but there are no toxic look-alikes.

Recipe: **Wood Sorrel Gimlet**

Ingredients

Base Syrup:

1 cup wood sorrel, chopped

1 cup water

1 cup sugar

Gimlet:

½ cup wood sorrel leaves, partially crushed

2 ounces gin

½ ounce lemon juice

1 ounce sorrel syrup

Method:

Simmer base ingredients in a saucepan for twenty minutes, cool. Blend Gimlet ingredients, except crushed sorrel leaves with crushed ice. Put sorrel in the bottom of a glass, add blended mixture and stir slightly.

CHAPTER THIRTY-SIX:

SUSTAINABLE STORAGE METHODS

FOR LONG-TERM USE OF HERBS

There is not the same abundance of wild fresh herbs all year round in northern latitudes, and sometimes when you pick herbs you might pick more than you can eat.

In this chapter, we will explore some of the easiest, most common, and low-budget preservation methods. This helps you to keep your wild herbs for extended periods of time.

Drying, freezing, and canning your herbs are the three most common ways to preserve them. However, they also may be preserved using oils and vinegars, or made into emulsions.

If you adhered to this guide, you spent a good deal of time getting ready to forage, learning the safety issues, how to identify plants, and which plants to pick. You may have discovered that there was far more required of you while foraging than you may have at first believed. You may also have found that you either loved being in nature, or you disliked it.

Now, you face the next set of tasks: preparing your foods and storing them. Like learning how to harvest, this step requires patience and knowledge, but it is very rewarding.

There is nothing that compares to the taste of a fresh wild berry dessert on a cold winter day, if the berries have been preserved properly. The lively taste of culinary herbs, frozen and then thawed to use in your favorite recipe, is far more exciting to the taste buds than store-bought cultivated herbs that may have been on the shelf for upwards of a year or more.

In other chapters, we learned about identification, how and where to forage, data on specific common plants, and a few recipes for each. In this chapter, we focus on sustainably storing your herbs. "Sustainably" is a keyword! Some ignore that vital aspect of herbalism.

Al learned about honey mushrooms from a friend, tasted a sample, and loved them. Immediately, he set out to harvest them in the campground where he and his friend summered. Since these mushrooms grow in clumps, he was able to slice off huge handfuls at a time. Within an hour, he had harvested six plastic bags full of the golden treats, clearing out the entire growth he had found nearby.

That night, he cooked a full bag to enjoy with his wife, and they washed down their feast with a bottle of wine. He paid the price for his greed and lack of knowledge. Both he and his wife suffered terrible stomachaches through the night and the next day. He did not know that this species reacted negatively with the consumption of alcohol!

He then washed and froze the remaining bags. During the winter, he discovered that those mushrooms also require special storage, and he was left with rubbery, tasteless, and useless frozen honey mushrooms. He had wasted nature's bounty, depriving others of the chance to harvest and enjoy them.

This book is presented in a manner that, we hope, you will find very easy to follow. Using the acronym "F.R.E.S.H.S." you have discovered how to **F**orage, how to do so **R**isk-free, how to identify **E**dible **S**pecies of **H**erbs, and now, how to **S**tore **S**ustainably.

But are you fully ready and eager to continue with your wildcrafting experience? If you are not enjoying and embracing that hobby, perhaps you should re-evaluate. The following brief exercise is intended to help you see if you want to continue. Preserving herbs takes effort and care. Are you ready and willing to take on that challenge? Let us find out.

We taught you about identifying and harvesting thirty-two common herbs. How many were you able to find and harvest? What difficulties did you experience?

EXERCISE

Foraging in the wild takes effort. There are no sidewalks, no easy pathways. The effort can be strenuous, the days in the sun (or rain) long. But foraging for new, wild herbs can be a healthier option, a great hobby, and encourage creative cooking. It allows you to be more independent from the grocery store, costs less, replaces health supplements, and can involve the whole family. With those points in mind, let's see if you are ready to continue with this novel experience.

Questions:

1. Did you find the effort to be physically strenuous, or did you find it to be a pleasurable experience?

2. Were you able to identify and harvest enough herbs to feel that the effort was worthwhile?

3. Do you believe that you saved money by foraging?

4. Were you able to cook successfully with your herbs?

5. Did you use any herbs medicinally or for a minor health concern?

6. Did you forage with other people, and, if so, did it enhance the experience?

7. Will you be foraging again?

8. Will you be expanding your pantry of herbs that you harvest?

STORAGE OF HARVESTED HERBS

The primary focus when storing herbs should be on preserving the medicinal value of the herb so that the active ingredients are not excessively diminished. There are numerous methods for preparing and storing processed herbs, but the primary means of storing raw plants are: freezing, drying, refrigeration, frozen blends, vinegar, oils, and tinctures.

Drying

There are five main ways to dry herbs: sun drying, air drying, microwave drying, oven drying, and dehydration. Each has its own advantages and drawbacks. Herbs are dried in a variety of ways, depending on the part of the plant used. There are drawbacks to each method, as well as advantages.

Air drying is a preferred method, as it is cost effective, easy, and preserves more of the oils and nutrients in the herb. It also takes a lot longer and a lot more space, as screens require lots of room around them, and bunch drying requires a dedicated area where they will not be disturbed.

Sun drying is quick, so long as the area is calm and free of dust and relatively free of birds and bugs. However, more delicate plants and flowers do not dry well in the sun.

Microwave drying tends to break down the herb structure if done on a higher power level. It is also a two-stage process that requires monitoring, but it is the quickest method of drying.

Oven drying requires that you constantly monitor the herbs so that they do not dry too quickly and lose all food or medicinal value, or burn. This process is far from energy-efficient, but it is the second-quickest.

Dehydration is the third-faster (or third-slowest, depending on perspective). It is inexpensive and efficient. The cost, of course, is in the initial purchase of a dehydrator—$40 to $100. When filling the dehydrator, though, care must be taken to make sure all leaves are of the same density and consistency. Stems and roots do not dry well or quickly in a dehydrator.

A dehydrator is a quick and easy option for drying herbs, but has limited space on its multiple levels. Thicker leaves, such as basil, parsley, plantain, and leaves from shrubs should be dried in a dehydrator. Do not use a microwave if possible since, even at low power, the plants will cook a little, degrading the essential oils in them.

All the methods of drying are generally the easiest and immediate way to preserve your harvested herbs.

For all herbs, shake out and cleanse prior to dying to remove debris and insects. Be careful of introducing more moisture to your plants if you intend to dry them.

Air Drying

Arrange separated, delicate or plain leaves (not heavy leaves like some sorrels) loosely on a screen, and place the screen in an area where it will not be disturbed by insects, animals, wind, sun or rain. If you must use aluminum screens, turn the leaves more often, so that there is no risk of rusting or molding of the herbs as they dry. Place the screen so that air underneath moves freely. You should place the screen in an area where sunlight is minimal. You may stack the screen trays vertically, if you leave at least 12-18 inches between levels. Turn the leaves at least twice each day. If humidity will be high at night, bring the trays indoors.

Sun Drying

For roots and seeds, herbs can be dried in direct sunlight. Flowers and delicate parts cannot be sundried, as they will break down easily and not dry evenly and much of the nutrient value may be lost. Use trays similar to those used in air drying, and arrange them in direct sun but out of the wind and away from pests. Turn regularly and store by your preferred method (sun-dried fruits occasionally are stored in oils, vinegar, or other suspensions, or used in emulsification).

Oven Drying

Your oven or toaster oven needs to be set at its lowest temperature (200°F), as you do not want to cook the herbs, but merely dehydrate them. Lay out the leaves on a silicone tray and dry them for as long as three or four hours. You will not need to turn them, but, as they dry, they may crumble. For this reason, you should wrap your lower, empty tray in foil to catch the dropping leaf parts.

Do not use your convection function, as the breeze will scatter the leaves around the oven. If you do use the lowest temperature and do not have an oven with an open element or open flame or pilot, you may use a muslin cloth, but this is not advisable for safety considerations.

Microwave Drying

Microwaves all have air movement as products cook. Using paper towels is difficult, but possible. However, arranging leaves on a standard microwave tray does not dry them properly without the paper to absorb some of the moisture. Microwave a thin layer of leaves, sandwiched between or placed on layers of paper towels, for one or two minutes, at 100-200-watt settings (generally level two). This is only double the power of an old incandescent bulb. Then, remove and replace paper towels if needed, and microwave for an additional thirty seconds at a time until they are dry.

A problem with microwaving is that the leaves may feel dry when removed from the microwave, but once they have cooled, they may again feel moist. You may wish to finish the drying process by air drying.

Dehydrator

Dehydrators can be inexpensive and easy to use. They generally have three, four, or five levels on which you can place herb leaves, stems, and berries. Dehydrators are very efficient at drying berries. Stems and roots take a long time, but you may choose to partially dry the roots and then finish by air drying them on racks in a darkened room.

Spread your leaves on each tray, making sure they are not packed tightly together. The settings are automatic: once the trays are loaded and the cap and motor are in place, simply turn on the dehydrator and allow it to dry the herbs for up to twelve hours.

STORAGE OF DRIED HERBS

Whole herbs store best. If you are sure that the herbs plants will not be disturbed, hang them loosely in a dark, undisturbed place with low humidity. Moisture is the enemy of dried herbs. However, you still can store whole dried herbs safely in large paper bags, or in containers with paper towels to absorb any moisture.

Storing in glass jars with cork stoppers, or other types of sealed glass works best.

Make sure that each herb collection is labeled with the name and date that the herb was prepared. Check every few weeks for quality.

Once the leaves are thoroughly dry, crumble them and store them in airtight glass containers (preferably not plastic or metal, so taste transfer does not occur), in a dark, undisturbed room where the temperature is moderately cool and does not fluctuate. You may also use paper bags that you seal, but if any moisture remains, this will cause problems with the product. If possible, use an old onion bag, fine camping mesh bag, or similar porous material.

Where you can store the entire plant (or stems, leaves, and flowers), hang the plant in a calm, dry, shaded area (if outdoors) or a dark, well-ventilated, dry room for several days, by bunching them at the stem base and securing them with an elastic band.

When storing dried herbs (or even fresh, frozen) do not grind or crush them until needed. The flavors will last longer, as it does in coffee beans, if you do not break up the molecules and release the oils the herbs contain. Try to avoid soft plastics with fresh herbs, as the plastics will leech the oils out. Store all herbs away from light and heat, ideally in a cooler location.

Freezing and Refrigeration

Conventional home freezing is less efficient than the flash freezing methods employed by large fruit and vegetable producers that supply grocery stores. They use "flash freezing," which very quickly freezes produce in such a manner that the cells of ice are much smaller than the crystals formed by conventional, slow refrigerator freezing. However, we can approximate the freezing techniques to create a quality frozen product.

Herbs do not require the flash freezing that berries, meat, and vegetables require commercially. And many herbs are not suitable for freezing.

Freezing preserves the essential oils in herbs, which gives them much of their flavor. To freeze, rinse the plants, let them air dry briefly, remove the leaves and place them, separated, on a flat tray in the freezer unit. If available, use a screen, so that moisture can wick or drip away. Once the leaves have frozen, bag them, seal the bag, and put them back in the freezer. Handle them quickly so that they do not thaw again.

Several herbs can be stored for up to three weeks in the refrigerator. Rinse the herbs and let air dry for a short time. Snip the bottom of the stem, like you would do for flowers in a vase. Place the herbs, stem down, in a jar with water in it. Wrap a plastic baggie or plastic wrap loosely around the plants and store them in the refrigerator, changing the water daily. This technique is similar to rooting clippings, and will allow the plant to continue to grow a little. A teaspoon of sugar provides some nutrition, along with a crushed antacid (calcium), if storing the product for a longer time.

Hard herbs (those with a hard stem), like mints or sage, can be stored by rolling them in a damp towel and placing them in a perforated plastic bag in the fridge.

Some of the delicate herbs that do not tolerate cold, like lavender or basil, can be kept in a jar outside of the refrigerator.

Sunlight is the enemy of all fresh herbs, and even artificial light can work quickly to degrade the quality of your harvested herbs, so even herbs like lavender should not be stored where the light is bright or near heat.

To freeze herbs, break them apart, separating leaves, flowers, and stems. Rinse them in cold water, set out to dry for thirty minutes then place them on a cookie sheet or screen tray from an air fryer oven before placing in the freezer until solidly frozen.

Remove the tray and pack frozen leaves in freezer bags, remove air, and replace in the freezer.

An alternative is to chop the leaves coarsely, then place them in ice cube trays, fill with water and freeze. When completely frozen, remove ice cubes to freezer bags to store until needed.

Innovative ways to store fresh herbs: chop them and mix them in a blender with a carrier oil such as olive, grapeseed, almond, or avocado oil, then refrigerate in jars for up to six weeks.

Make butter by softening coconut oil, mix in generous amounts of your preferred herb leaves, blend, then solidify in butter dishes or containers in the fridge for up to two months. Alternatively, coconut oil, being a very viscous, dense oil, may be frozen once you have blended your herbs with it, and then you can use it as needed.

Lastly, purée your herbs with a little oil and freeze in plastic bags.

Canning and Other Storage Techniques

Root crops and other low acid, high-density plants can be canned by blanching for three minutes and sealing them in sterilized jars (in the same way as vegetables are canned). When canning herb leaves, use about one to one and a half cups of herbs per three cups of boiled water or vinegar and place them in jars, sealing them for later use. To extend life, keep the herbs stored in the refrigerator.

Peel or scrub roots before blanching. With thick roots, stems or bark, slice the root lengthwise.

Jams and jellies with fruits all follow a couple of basic recipe patterns, with the only variation being the type of jam being made. Moisture-rich jellies require slightly less liquid to be added, while pectin and gelatin provide the thickening agent. Apple juice, stevia (an herb), or sugar provide much of the sweetener.

Many fresh herbs can be stored by chopping the leaves (and roots, bark, or stems) coarsely, then storing them in carrier oils or in vinegar that has been heated.

Other, more temporary, storage techniques are infusions, tinctures, decoctions, distillations, liniments, ointments, creams, lotions, wines, syrups, and candies.

Equipment and Supplies Needed

The proper tools are as important to storing herbs as is the proper knowledge. We have compiled a list of essential tools that you will need for your storage project.

You will need, depending upon the storage method that you are using, the following supplies:

- strainer or sieve

- kitchen scissors

- good quality kitchen knife

- cutting board

- food grater

- dehydrator

- mesh oven trays

- screens or drying trays

- silicone cookie sheets

- blender

- microwave

- toaster oven

- mortar and pestle

- ice cube trays

- glass jars with cork or mason sealing lids

- vacuum bag sealing machine

- cool, dry dark storage area with shelving

- plastic freezer bags

- paper bags

- paper towels

- tea towels

- coffee bean grinder

- elastic bands

- twine

- pickling or white vinegar

- carrier oils such as olive, grapeseed, avocado or almond

- sugar

- pectin

- gelatin

Conclusion:
Forage Risk-Free for Edible
Species of Herbs, Sustainably

This book is about safely identifying edible species of wild plants that will complement your menu and your apothecary in a manner that is good for the environment.

Safety and sustainability are the two key takeaways for foragers as they begin exploring the world of wildcrafting.

We have provided information on thirty-two edible, wild plants, but this is minuscule compared to the number of species that you can harvest within a very small radius of where you live, wherever that may be in North America.

While many of these plants also grow in other regions of the world, you now have a decent list of local plants for your dinner plate or your medicine cabinet. Knowing where to find these plants, when to harvest, and how to harvest is the critical first step in your new hobby.

There are over 5,000 edible plants in North America alone. Do not expect that you will be able to identify most of them soon. Many foragers, after years of harvesting, may have only an array of fewer than one hundred herbs and spices, but they know the myriad ways that those plants can be used in culinary dishes, used to treat ailments, or used to keep you healthy.

It is better to know a few herbs intimately than know a little about many. It is better to harvest a small quantity and variety, while preserving the bulk for future harvesters than to gorge on the entire supply, only to have it disappear from the forests and fields.

Add a few herbs to your knowledge base every year and soon you will have a cornucopia of free, healthy, tasty food at your fingertips. Many of us complement our natural diet with a few store-bought items, rather than the other way around.

Rediscover the power of nature and the energy of healthy eating as you interact with the outdoors. Just the experience could add years to your life!

Even if you chose to merely step into nature and learn about the plants around you, without harvesting, you will be richer for it. You don't need to be an expert at the start, and you don't need to be an expert at the end. You just need to embrace the natural world and appreciate what it offers, and you will be enriched for it.

Just follow the F.R.E.S.H.S. steps to identifying and enjoying your wild herbal garden. Foraging properly and safely, taking the time to become intimate with this wild world around you, and practicing mindfulness in your harvesting helps to make you a part of the raw, organic world around you. That, on its own, is a giant step toward healthy living.

Nearly ten percent of all plants, worldwide, are edible. Over thousands of years, people have come to understand and embrace their value for cooking and for medicinal purposes. More importantly, perhaps, they have recognized how intertwined we humans are with the natural world, and how essential each herb is to us.

Nearly every edible plant has its own story. Throughout history, folklore connects each valuable herb with the gods of the era and of that civilization, yet, almost universally and independently, each of those herbs has been attributed with the same healing powers. This occurred, even though those cultures were sometimes thousands of miles apart.

The stories and myths that plants possess may not have a base in scientific fact, but the aura that surrounds each specimen is almost godlike, acknowledging the supernatural power of plants.

As you forage, pay tribute to those gods. Do not pillage the bounty over which they preside. Believe, or be skeptical of the myths, fables, and lore. Recognize that, should you destroy the natural wonder of the world over which the gods preside, they will exact their revenge. We cannot afford to risk losing this wondrous environment.

GLOSSARY OF TERMS

Anthelmintic: expelling or destroying parasitic worms, especially of the intestine.

Antibacterial: intended to kill or reduce the harmful effects of bacteria, especially when used on the skin.

Anti-carcinogenic: that which protects against carcinogens.

Antidepressant: a drug used to reduce feelings of sadness and worry.

Antidiabetic: that which protects against diabetes.

Antihistamine: a type of drug that is used to treat medical conditions caused by an extreme or regular allergic reaction to particular substances.

Antihypertensive: abnormally high blood pressure and especially arterial blood pressure.

Anti-inflammatory: an anti-inflammatory drug is one that is used to reduce pain and swelling.

Antimicrobial: any agent that kills or suppresses the growth of microorganisms.

Antipruritic: tending to relieve or prevent itching.

Antiseptic: Substance that prevents or arrests the growth or action of microorganisms by inhibiting their activity or by destroying them.

Antiviral: an antiviral drug or treatment cures an infection or disease caused by a virus.

Cephalic: of or relating to the head.

Choleretic: promoting bile secretion by the liver.

Coagulant: the process of becoming viscous or thickened into a coherent mass.

Decongestant: a medicine that helps you to breathe more easily, especially if you have a cold.

Deobstruent: removing obstructions; having the power to clear or open the natural ducts of the fluids and secretions of the body; aperient.

Detoxifier: to remove a harmful substance (such as a poison or toxin) or the effect of such a substance from something.

Disinfectant: an agent used to disinfect something.

Depurative: purification of impurities or heterogeneous matter.

Expectorant: a type of cough medicine used to make phlegm less thick in the lungs.

Irritant: something that irritates or excites.

Phytoestrogenic: pertaining to a chemical compound (such as genistein) that occurs naturally in plants and has estrogenic properties.

Progesteronic: relating to a female steroid sex hormone.

Testosteronic: relating to a hormone that is a hydroxysteroid ketone that is responsible for inducing and maintaining male secondary sex characters.

Vaso Protector: a treatment that protects the vascular system.

THE HOLISTIC BOOK OF HERBAL MEDICINE & NATURAL REMEDIES

INTRODUCTION

"The healing comes from nature and not from the physician. Therefore, the physician must start from nature with an open mind."

-by Paracelsus

Have you ever wondered why you see so many pharmaceutical ads on television? What do they have to gain? Many people use prescription and non-prescription pain medications for a variety of reasons. For example, if you or a loved one is suffering from pain or chronic discomfort, you might be tempted to reach for over-the-counter drugs like Ibuprofen or Acetaminophen. But these drugs often aren't strong enough to provide the relief that many people need, so they turn to prescription opioids.

In the late 1990s, pharmaceutical companies persuaded doctors that opioid painkillers would not lead to addiction, and doctors began prescribing them at increased rates. In 2017, the United States was in an opioid epidemic. Over 33,000 Americans died from drug overdoses that year alone, which is just the tip of the iceberg.

One of the primary tactics used by pharmaceutical corporations to increase their profits is to sponsor ad campaigns that convince people to abuse–or make liberal use of– prescription painkillers. As a result, many people have become hooked on opioids after years of being prescribed them legitimately.

But opioids are highly addictive and come with a host of severe side effects, including overdose, digestive problems, weakened immune systems, depression, anxiety, suicidal thoughts, and more. Many addicts who can't access prescription painkillers turn to heroin. The illegal nature of this substance only adds to the problem because people who buy it on the streets often don't know exactly what they're purchasing and may be vulnerable to dangerous contaminants like fentanyl or carfentanil, which are potent opioids and can be deadly.

The opioid pandemic that has gripped the United States is the product of aggressive and deceitful marketing by pharmaceutical firms and doctors.

According to the Centers for Disease Control and Prevention (CDC), from 1999 to 2017, there were over 183,000 deaths from prescription opioid overdoses. This is more than the combined four-decade homicide count in the United States (192,369) and Iraq (182,965). It also eclipses the number of deaths from illegal drugs, like cocaine (41,386), methamphetamines (28,865), and heroin (15,482) over the same period.

The pharmaceutical companies made false claims regarding opioids and how they treat pain. They have repeatedly been incorrect, resulting in the deaths of millions of individuals from opioid-related disorders and diseases.

It is not the first time pharmaceuticals have significantly harmed public health to increase profits. In the 1990s, pharmaceutical companies were responsible for approximately 60% of all deaths due to overdose—primarily illegal opiate painkillers such as OxyContin.

Some of the significant 'pharma' scandals in history (EcoWatch, 2022):

1. Phenylpropanolamine (PPA)

Phenylpropanolamine, also known as "the coffee pill," is a stimulant drug used by millions of people every day. It was first sold by the pharmaceutical company Smith Kline Beecham in 1937 and later by the British pharmaceutical company GlaxoSmithKline (GSK).

After over 60 years in use, the FDA issued a public health advisory in 2001 warning that PPA could cause serious harm to the heart and other parts of the body, and this was primarily because of its effect on blood pressure. In August 2000, the FDA gave GSK 60 days to provide data that showed that PPA benefits outweighed its risks.

In March 2001, GSK voluntarily removed PPA from the market after it was found that there were no data available to show how safe it was.

These are just a few of the most notable scandals in the history of prescription drugs. This should give you a clue of how difficult it is for the FDA and other regulatory bodies to track what happens inside the pharmaceutical industry.

Almost every year, there are reports of fresh scandals related to prescription drugs with harmful side effects and other negative consequences.

2. Diethylstilbestrol (DES)

Diethylstilbestrol, or DES, is a synthetic estrogen manufactured by the US pharmaceutical company Eli Lilly and Co., and a host of other companies around the world. It was used in the United States from 1939 until 1971 to treat pregnant women with "generalized preeclampsia" at 40 or more weeks.

In 1959, DES was used to treat 11,000 pregnant women in France. Some of these women gave birth to daughters who later developed severe congenital disabilities. In 1970, the Food and Drug Administration of the United States (FDA) concluded that treating pregnant women with DES resulted in a small increase in the risk of miscarriage for these women.

Despite this, DES was still widely used until 1975, when it was withdrawn from the market because of its potential to cause "genetic damage" to the unborn children of exposed mothers. The mothers had no idea that this was taking place.

The FDA was heavily criticized for failing to warn the public about the risk of adverse effects due to using DES while pregnant. The scandal is known by many as "the most shameful moment in the agency's history."

3. Thalidomide

Thalidomide was a drug that was produced by the German company Chemie Grünenthal. It was first approved for use in West Germany in 1956 and then quickly released worldwide, In the United Kingdom, France, and Canada. This drug was known as Contergan, which later became a useful synonym for "terrible" or "a disaster." Within weeks of its release, Thalidomide had affected thousands of babies.

Thalidomide was heavily promoted as a safe, effective way to combat morning sickness during pregnancy—an approach that was widely accepted at the time. It was sold over the counter and had no clear label instructions. As a result, pregnant mothers began to take this drug daily.

The discovery of thalidomide's terrible effects was slow. Still, once it became clear that it caused congenital disabilities and other related health issues, the drug was taken off the market and quickly replaced by safer options. In 1961, Grünenthal offered a payment of 2 million Deutschmarks to cover any legal expenses of children born with defects and their care costs.

However, this was not enough, and the company was forced to pay out more money to settle further claims. In total, they paid more than $21 million in compensation. The number of lawsuits totaled approximately 6,000—making it one of the biggest pharmaceutical scandals ever.

4. Terfenadine (Seldane)

Terfenadine, made by Hoechst Marion Roussel (now Aventis), was first approved by the FDA in 1986 and was quickly purchased by Smith Kline Beecham. It had already become a bestseller by this time. Smith Kline Beecham claimed that it was safe for children and senior citizens up to 55 years—even though it had never been tested on these groups.

In May 1997, after over 3 million people had reportedly taken Seldane, eight patients reported seizures after taking one pill per day for at least two weeks. In 1998, the FDA ordered a recall of terfenadine in all doses. It was also banned in the European Union following a report on the risk of heart attacks.

Terfenadine was eventually replaced by a new drug called Prilosec. Smith Kline Beecham subsequently pleaded guilty to criminal charges concerning their drug marketing— although they were not required to pay any penalties.

5. Fenfluramine/phentermine (Fen-Phen)

Fenfluramine and phentermine are appetite suppressants, commonly sold as the most common drug to lose weight. In 1992, the FDA recalled these drugs after researchers found that they could cause heart valve problems and sudden death in mice if they were given high doses. They were also proven to cause liver damage in humans when taken daily.

Wyeth-Ayerst Laboratories' manufacturer denied a link between the drug and heart problems. The company also claimed that the studies had been misinterpreted and that the drugs were safe to use. However, their claims were later proved to be false. In 1997, a study found a significant increase in the risk of heart attack if a person took these drugs instead of dieting or exercising.

6. Vioxx

Vioxx was a prescription painkiller produced by Merck & Co., a leading pharma company that manufactures various drugs, including antibiotics and vaccines. The FDA approved it in 1999 for use as a non-steroidal anti-inflammatory drug (NSAID). The drug was notorious for causing severe health problems, including heart attacks, kidney failure, lung problems, and strokes. According to some estimates, Merck & Co.'s sales of Vioxx totaled $4 billion between 1999 and 2004.

In 2004, Merck & Co. faced a wave of lawsuits from individual plaintiffs, who claimed that they had suffered severe health issues after taking Vioxx. They eventually settled with over 100,000 people.

In 2005, Merck & Co. agreed to pay about $4.85 billion for criminal and civil wrongdoing and compensate people who suffered from Vioxx side effects. This is one of the largest pharmaceutical scandals ever.

If you're reading this book, there's a good chance you take at least one prescription drug—or maybe even several—every day and don't realize how dangerous it may be. This point should be stressed because it is crucial to remember that you are already potentially causing your body harm by taking the wrong drug.

You should be aware that pharmaceutical companies significantly influence how drugs are approved by regulatory bodies and marketed to the public. As we've seen above, there is ample evidence indicating that many free prescription drug samples (such as those offered at retail pharmacies) may cause significant harm. This is because many of these sample medications have unknown adverse effects.

You may be practicing a healthy lifestyle and getting plenty of exercise, but chances are very high that you are not getting enough information about prescription drugs in the media. This means that you are likely to be ignorant about the potential side effects of some medicines that you take.

You must understand that modern medicine is not a science—it's a profession. This means that, like any other profession (lawyers, mechanics, etc.), it relies mainly on trust to function well.

Using natural medicines that have been both proven and studied is an entirely different story. People who use these types of natural treatments are more likely to trust them than those who abuse prescription drugs—because they know they can take charge of their health.

This book will give you the steps to get into Herbal Medicine following the **HEALING** framework.

HEALING stands for:

- **H**ave a good grasp of herbs

- **E**nsure your safety

- **A**cquire your herbs

- **L**earn the methods of preparation

- **I**dentify what you need

- **N**ow start concocting

- **G**et comfortable with formulation

Each step will be covered in its chapter and will detail what you need to do and consider. This book should teach you the fundamentals of Herbal Medicine. This means you can't use this book as a reference for every situation that comes up in your life. You need to use it as a baseline and then look into specific conditions or issues and individual ingredients that you need.

The two most important points about starting your journey with herbs are to ensure that you don't take any herbs without first knowing what they are and how to use them. This means that you must identify the herbs you want to use before you go out and buy them, ensuring your safety. Some herbs are more dangerous, but you can quickly identify those and look for safe ones.

The second important point is to ensure that you acquire a good quantity of the herbs you want to use. Find out what quantity or amount you will need. This will only take a small amount of time if you have a little knowledge about the herb in question, as well as about what it does for your body.

Once you have acquired the correct herbs, it's time to start preparing them. This is easily done by following the methods of preparation given in the book. After that, you can start identifying what you need. You may have a condition that will require multiple herbs or one herb for two different situations.

Learning how to concoct your own herbal medicine is one of the essential points in this book. We prioritize our health

205

by eating right and regularly exercising. You may already be trying to shift to a more plant-based lifestyle through the foods you eat and the products you use, but how do you deal with those various ailments like a cold, a wound, or a headache? You don't have to grab that cough syrup or Tylenol. It's possible to create your remedies so you know exactly what you're putting into your body.

Who is Small Footprint Press?

Small Footprint Press, established amidst the pandemic, is a self-publishing company of experts that aims to promote sustainable survival—equipping you to live a sustainable, conscious, and independent lifestyle to make the world a better place for yourself and future generations to come.

As the world progresses, we believe that the importance of sustainable survival becomes more and more clear. Our planet faces various challenges, including climate change, dwindling resources, population growth, and pandemics. To secure a bright future for our children, *now* is the time we must take steps to save our planet.

We accomplish this by simply empowering you to prepare for potential disasters for yourself and your loved ones. Gone are the days when you stress about the day of the unknown!

Our books are a collaboration of different authors, each with their perspective and expertise. This makes for a well-rounded book that covers various topics in-depth, ensuring the highest quality standards. It also makes for a more engaging read, as each author brings their style to the table.

Similarly, orchestras are made up of different instruments, each with its unique sound and purpose. Once these instruments play as one in harmony, the result is extraordinary.

We believe that one way to bridge a community of people with a shared purpose and values is through books! In this community, you build genuine relationships, share similar experiences, and be empowered to take action.

You are not alone. There's something special about a journey taken with others. Whether exploring a new city or embarking on a long hike, sharing the experience with others makes you enjoy the journey more than the destination.

So allow us to join you in your journey to a compelling life of sustainable survival!

Interested in joining our cause? Download your FREE resources at the beginning of the book!

Chapter One:
What We Get Wrong About
Herbal Medicine

The term herbal medicine seems straightforward. What makes herbs medicinal? How did we learn to use them?

A lot of plants can be used medicinally. Each part of a plant can help heal different ailments, from the roots to the treetops. Plants contain chemicals that have positive, negative, or neutral effects on the body.

For example, most parts of the deadly nightshade (belladonna), as the name might suggest, are very toxic and were used as a poison in folklore. However, the leaves and roots of the plant can be used as a muscle relaxant and for peptic ulcers. So, this plant has both positive and negative aspects. Despite how interesting it sounds, do not take deadly nightshade unless it's prescribed to you. An overdose can be fatal. If taken in the correct dosage, the plants with positive aspects are used for herbal medicine and the basis for modern medicine.

Beyond simply plants grown for herbal use, many plants we eat are also effective for herbal medicine. If you've ever lived outside of Western nations, in Africa, Asia or elsewhere, you may be familiar with fruits and vegetables consumed for specific illnesses.

Papaya, for example, is not just a delicious fruit for snacking on but is also used for deworming, digestive issues, and healing wounds. Foods that double as medicine in the US include oats, lemons, onions, and garlic. These are foods quickly and inexpensively found in grocery stores across the US, and they each have beneficial uses and are great to have on hand. So herbal medicine can include edible plants and herbal plants.

Today, roughly 11% of the medications classified as "basic" or "essential" by the World Health Organization originated in flowering plants, with many more coming from non-flowering plants. Everything from aspirin to quinine, digitalis to morphine began as a natural substance taken from plants. And this is only the start. Many plants have leaves, flowers, roots, and fruits that can treat or prevent various ailments.

Plants have been used to heal humans from the beginning of time, and we can use them to heal ourselves. Our bodies are organisms that live and breathe and are constantly striving for homeostasis. The systems of the body have natural mechanisms to maintain balance and can often react against us, including the immune system.

An immune system is a group of cells that help defend your body by fighting infections, healing damaged tissue, and developing disease resistance. Herbal medicines can help keep our immune systems in good shape.

Before being approved, any medicine derived from plants prescribed by a medical expert has typically undergone years of rigorous research into efficacy and safety. In truth, only a tiny percentage of medications are approved by the FDA.

What about plant-based vitamins and minerals? There hasn't been enough research to determine their efficacy and safety. However, there is enough evidence to show that they can be used safely.

On Thursday, April 4, 2001, actress Suzanne Somers stated that she had treated her breast cancer using Iscador. Iscador is a natural medicine made by extracting mistletoe. The mistletoe plant has been known to have healing powers, which Somers tried after her diagnosis with breast cancer.

Somers took her doctor's advice and had a malignant lump removed, followed by radiation therapy, to eradicate any leftover cancer. Sandi Mendelson, her publicist, said she was taking Iscador to enhance her immune system.

For 25 years, Somers has practiced alternative medicine—acupuncture, therapeutic massage, biofeedback, and using vitamins. Somers also said she lives a very healthy lifestyle with lots of exercise.

Do these alternative treatments work?

According to Somers, Iscador has helped her with energy and stamina, and she admits that the herb has made a real difference.

Somers is not alone. Alternative medicines are used by many people who have been diagnosed with cancer to supplement established therapy.

"I'm thrilled using both," she said. "It's worked for me."

The majority of herbs may be found in health food stores in your area and online herbal shops, and some herbs can be found in your backyard or a nearby forest.

What Is Herbalism?

Herbalism is the practice of using herbal/plant medicines to treat and prevent disease. These medicines should be held in the highest level of respect because they are natural remedies derived from plants. Herbal medicines can be any part of a plant, whether a leaf, root, bark, or fruit. Herbalism is practiced worldwide, and it has been used for thousands of years by tribal people like ourselves.

Learning about herbal medicine could be a satisfying experience; therefore, here are some tips for safely harvesting wild plants—for the plants, for the cultivators, and for the ecology in which they live.

What Are Medicinal Herbs?

Herbs are found naturally throughout the world. They grow everywhere; they could be in your backwoods, in your backyard, or even alongside the road. Where plants thrive, you are likely to find herbs or a perfect habitat for growing them.

Herbs are organized into various groups depending on their properties. For example, some herbs are considered culinary herbs used to flavor food, while others are deemed aromatic herbs and add fragrance. Medicinal herbs are grouped for their properties that can be used for medicinal purposes.

Medicinal herbs can be a wide variety of plant types. Medicinal herbs can be sun-loving, shade-loving, herbaceous, woody, perennial, or annual. The plant parts containing the medicinal properties are general. People routinely use all the functions described below. You have probably been using herbal medicine for a long time without even knowing it. If you have ever used herbs such as basil, mint, peppermint, sage, thyme, and rosemary for adding great flavors to your food—then you have already been practicing herbal medicine.

Common culinary herbs and spices have many medicinal properties and can also be considered medicinal herbs. We can find numerous others in our kitchen which have been used for medicinal purposes, such as salves, teas, poultices, and more. You can also find many more common medicinal herbs in food that you buy from the store. For example, cabbage can be used as an effective poultice for hives or shingles, and horseradish is a beautiful sinus infection home treatment.

Okay, you may be thinking that those are not medicinal herbs; they are vegetables. However, any plant with healing properties is regarded as a medicinal herb.

Herbalism has been evolving for many centuries around the needs of people. So, wouldn't it make sense to use readily available things? The truth is this: for the most part, the most common plants make the most effective home remedies for common ailments.

How does herbal medicine differ from conventional medicine?

Conventional medicine is the more modern and scientific form of medicine. They focus on drugs, surgical procedures, and other procedures to target a specific problem or ailment.

Herbal medicine involves using botanical extracts and drugs. It focuses on ideal health and well-being through herbs, tinctures, poultices, teas, oils, etc. It looks at nutritional needs first before moving on to issues with the body, such as infections, allergies, obesity, etc.

Herbal medicine is a very appropriate form of treatment for people looking for alternative treatment methods. The beneficial properties are organic; they run through the body and heal what needs healing, more effectively than any pharmaceutical drug could.

Western Herbal Medicine

Western herbal therapy treats the whole individual rather than trying to address each symptom alone. The approach entails a detailed clinical assessment. The clinical evaluation includes a history of the presenting illness, what the patient has already done to treat their condition, symptoms present in the body, previous diagnoses, and treatment plans. It's critical to know what has and hasn't worked for you in the past to comprehend your condition entirely. This will give Western herbalists a clear picture of what to do next. The herbalist looks at your:

- Diet

- Family history

- Lifestyle

- Personal health history

Western herbalists typically use European and North American herbs to create their medications. They also employ Chinese and Indian herbs and spices.

Traditional Chinese Medicine (TCM)

TCM is widely used in China and throughout Asia. TCM focuses on using herbs to maintain health and prevent illness. They look at the patient's energy levels, emotional well-being, diet, lifestyle, etc. They seek to balance all of these factors through herbal medicines.

Typically, TCM focuses on using five plant categories:

1. Wood (metabolism),

2. Fire (heat),

3. Earth (bio-mineral),

4. Metal (essence), and

5. Water (moisture).

These categories focus on the individual's health benefits and determine the type of medicine they would like to use.

TCM's purpose is to restore your Qi's balance (pronounced chee). Qi is the energy that flows through your body. TCM practitioners believe that if your Qi is balanced and flowing correctly, all of your organs will work properly, and you will be well and happy. TCM focuses on the following:

- Massage therapy

- Herbal remedies

- Tai chi, a set of movement exercises (pronounced tie chee)

- Acupuncture

- Qi gong is a type of traditional Chinese breathing and movement practice (pronounced chee gong)

TCM uses herbal remedies and traditional Chinese medicines; practitioners also make use of western medication. Some TCM practitioners will create specific formulas for you to take to treat a particular ailment.

Why do Cancer Patients use Herbal Medicine?

Herbal medicines are a powerful tool in cancer treatment. According to the American Cancer Society, nearly 70% of patients with cancer use some form of complementary therapy. The most common form is herbal medicine, followed by homeopathy and Chinese herbal medicine. Herbal medicine has been used for over 6,000 years across many cultures and continents. Studies have shown that many herbs can help to fight cancer. Some have anti-cancer properties, while others help prevent cancer from causing harm to the body.

Herbal medicine can be used alongside conventional therapies. Herbs are used to treat the body and help the body heal itself, and they are applied topically to affect the lymph nodes, organs, or subtle channels that run through the body.

The uses of herbal medicine are not limited to cancer patients, though. Many people use these remedies because they offer so many benefits for overall health and well-being and a way to manage certain physical conditions such as arthritis or high blood pressure or even conditions like insomnia and anxiety.

Benefits of Herbal Medicine

You only need to visit a couple of shops to see countless herbal or all-natural products, in addition to dietary supplements and herbal medicine solutions. So, when did this herbal movement begin?

Herbal medicine is ancient, and let's just say we wouldn't have gotten where we are as a species without it. If it weren't for herbal medicine, our life span would be 30 years or less.

Herbal medicine has helped us heal ailments and injuries and, therefore, live longer.

Folklore and generational knowledge evolved over the centuries to become traditional medicine in different regions. In the West (Europe and settled North America), herbal medicine evolved from the writings of Greek physicians, but by that point, China and India already had established herbal treatments that are still used today. So, when you practice herbal medicine, you are continuing the traditions of our ancestors and reinforcing the bond between humans and nature.

Today, herbal medicine is having a resurgence in the West, though it has always been around in other areas of the world. In countries where malaria is common, many communities use herbal remedies when more modern medicine isn't available. Unfortunately, modern medicine is starting to fail us in treating certain diseases.

Many of our diseases adapt to modern medicine, specifically antibiotics, and are becoming resistant to them. In cases like this, herbal medicine can be used to help. Using more herbal medicines instead of relying on synthetic ones can help to ensure that diseases are treated, even if they are medicine-resistant.

Therefore, when it comes to choosing which products to buy, it is essential to understand how they are made and precisely what their active ingredients are.

Should you encounter any impacts you did not expect from utilizing a herb, then it is likely because of the total dosage required, you have overindulged. Any discomfort is short-term; only the time it requires the chemicals to depart from your system. One guideline: if you are allergic to some plant, herb, or spice, then you are allergic to the essential oils, also, and potentially related plant species.

Affordability

Modern medicine has been great for the overall health of humanity. Still, things are becoming more expensive, getting medical care is more complicated for many individuals than for others, and large numbers of people cannot afford it. Using herbs as natural remedies enable you to save your hard-earned money.

Saving money may not be possible with pharmaceutical medicines, given their typically high cost. Aside from being the more affordable solution for ailments, botanical remedies are often equally effective compared to drug-based medications.

Herbal medicine is also one of the most cost-effective ways to improve your health and save on healthcare expenses. Purchasing herbal supplements from the store is far less expensive than paying for doctor visits and medications. Herbal medicine is even more inexpensive and cost-effective when growing your herbs and making home remedies.

You'll be surprised at how much pleasure, ease, and money you can save by making your teas, salves, syrups, tinctures, and capsules, mainly if you use herbs you've cultivated yourself. Making simple herbal home remedies for coughs, sprains, and infections is the ideal place to start. They are not only practical, but they can also save you money on family healthcare.

Efficacy of Treatment

Many herbal medicines have gone through numerous trials, which have helped confirm their efficacy to help ensure that they are safe for use.

Immune-Boosting Properties

Herbal medicine helps to improve immune function such that it does not interfere with the body's physiological processes; instead, it supports the body and helps keep those processes going. Every aspect of the body is boosted to the point that it suddenly gets a lift and can function to its fullest.

Native North America is another one of the birthplaces of herbal medicine, and their relationship with nature was strong enough to make them understand the benefits of the herbs and plants around them. This connection has been translated to many locations of the world, making their remedies more widely used by people today.

Herbal medicine has numerous advantages and can improve our lives and health in various ways. One of the most evident benefits of taking herbal medications is that they can help to boost health and improve the immune system. This is an invisible aspect of our health.

Growing our herbs and making our medicines to treat ourselves and our families takes very little time, effort, or money. Herbal medicine is one of the most natural, affordable, accessible, and effective self-treatments and care methods.

Another great benefit of herbal medicine is that there are relatively few side effects. While people have adverse reactions to specific herbs and foods, this is not because of the plants being toxic, but rather an individual response.

This does not mean that no toxic plants can cause adverse reactions; however, such plants are illegal and are not included in herbal home remedies. The herbs used in home remedies have been used for centuries as both medicine and food with little to no side effects.

Such side effects may include nausea, upset stomach, sore throat, a skin rash, or itchy eyes. Generally, the side effects do not last long and will disappear after discontinuing the use of that particular herb.

Different Health and Medical Concerns that Herbal Medicine Addresses

All the functions described below are routinely used by people to maintain health and treat disease symptoms. There is a substantial amount of scientific and clinical data in support of the use of botanical medicines in each of these conditions. Each of these principles is discussed further in the sections that follow.

Cardiovascular and Circulatory Functions

Clinical research suggests that botanical medications can be used to maintain cardiovascular and circulatory health and to treat cardiovascular disorders like arrhythmia and moderate hypertension (or high blood pressure). Here are some examples:

- Hawthorn

- Garlic

- Ginkgo

- Echinacea

- Ginseng

The Cardiovascular System is a complex system of vessels, valves, and muscles that carries blood throughout the body. To maintain cardiovascular health, it's crucial to support its smooth and regular flow. Heart-healthy botanical medications — like garlic, ginkgo, and echinacea — can be used to help support the cardiovascular system in three significant ways:

1. Antiarrhythmic, with significant evidence to demonstrate that they can reduce the frequency of the irregular heartbeat

2. Cardiovascular protection, with studies showing a significant decrease in heart attacks after using these compounds

3. Anti-inflammatory, with studies showting the potential benefits of botanical medications for reducing inflammation throughout the body.

Digestive, Gastrointestinal, and Liver Functions

Herbal medicines used in the gastrointestinal and liver systems can be used to maintain digestive health and treat gastrointestinal disorders. Some of these common side effects include stomachaches, acid indigestion, and heartburn. Here are some examples:

- Peppermint

- Ginger

- Fennel

- Dong Quai

In the gastrointestinal system, our bodies process food to produce energy and create waste products through a series of physiological processes that are controlled by hormones. The gut also acts as a barrier to protect our internal organs.

In some cases, the gastrointestinal system can be compromised by stress or disease. Botanical medications can be used to support the digestive process and help treat health conditions like nausea, vomiting, and diarrhea.

Endocrine and Hormonal Functions

Healing through the endocrine system can take place through the glands, also known as endocrine glands. When these glands are damaged or malfunctioning, they can cause problems throughout your body. Proper endocrine function is crucial to maintaining proper metabolism and balance throughout the body.

Endocrine disorders may involve hormonal imbalances, such as low thyroid function, which may result in weight gain or loss, pain, and fatigue. Additionally, the substances below are used to restore hormone balance and repair hormone dysfunction in both men and women. Some common hormonal disorders that herbal medicine may help with include:

- Andropause, or the aging male syndrome, is a decrease in testosterone levels in men that may occur between the ages of 40–60

- Menopausal symptoms and premenstrual syndrome (PMS) in women

- Low Estrogen in women

Herbal medicines may also be used to support healthy endocrine function and promote hormone balance. Some of the most often utilized herbs for endocrine disorders are listed below:

- Dong Quai

- Andrographis

- Ginseng

- Dandelion

- Schisandra

Genito-urinary and Renal Functions

Urinary tract infections (UTIs) come in a variety of forms that can affect the urinary system. Symptoms may include burning or pain during urination, cloudy urine, or blood in the urine. These conditions can be caused by a variety of factors, including infection with bacteria or yeast, urine blockage due to kidney stones, and irritation to the bladder or urethra. Herbal medicines used in the genito-urinary and renal systems can address these conditions by dealing with the underlying cause of UTIs as well as the symptoms associated with them.

Herbal medicine can also be used to maintain healthy kidney function and reduce kidney problems caused by diabetes, infection, or kidney failure. Here are some examples:

- Garlic

- Parsley

- Uva Ursi

- Cranberry

Herbal remedies may be used to treat genito-urinary and renal systems disorders like bladder and urinary infection, cystitis, kidney stones, excessive bleeding from the bladder or prostate, as well as urge incontinence. Kidney failure and chronic kidney disease can be treated using herbal medication because of its antioxidant effect on the kidneys. Many herbs reduce protein in the urine, which is a complication of kidney failure.

Reproductive Functions

Herbal medicines can assist in the treatment of reproductive system disorders, pain, disease, and support fertility. These include:

- Treating menopausal and PMS symptoms. The most well-studied herbal drugs for menopausal symptoms are black cohosh, agnes vitex/chasteberry, and sage. Numerous clinical trials have shown that black cohosh, specifically, works as well as hormone replacement therapy for the treatment of menopause symptoms and other conditions (De Smet, 2004;

Ebeling et al., 2006). While data show that black cohosh appears to be safe, there are insufficient data on its long-term efficacy (Ebeling et al., 2006).

Preliminary studies suggest that St. John's wort may be effective in treating premenstrual syndrome (PMS) (Eisinger et al. 2003).

- Managing pregnancy. According to clinical studies, ashwagandha may be effective in treating morning sickness in early pregnancy (Kaur et al., 2006; Sukumar & Chauhan, 2002).

- Treating sexual dysfunction. According to clinical studies, extracts of the root of the ginseng plant (Panax Ginseng) improve male sexual function. Ginseng also relieves symptoms in post-menopausal women and men with impotence (Sakamoto et al., 2001).

These are just a few examples of functions. The list is endless.

Since plants contain a considerable array of different chemical substances, an attempt to categorize all their possible functions would be futile. The one-to-one correspondence between a "disease" and its "cure" will never hold water for all human complex disorders, and also not for many minor ailments. Even when herbs provide relief from symptoms of disease, this may not mean that they can cure diseases in the conventional sense of the word.

Applications of Herbal Medicine

Unlike Somers, most people with cancer use herbal medicine to manage pain and deal with anxiety and depression, not as an immunity booster that helps to fight tumors.

Herbal medicine is used to help with the following:

- Hay fever

- Irritable bowel syndrome

- Menstrual problems

- Eczema, and many other low-grade but persistent issues.

Stress is a constant part of daily life in the United States, so stress relief can be a significant benefit of using herbal medicine. Herbs–even the act of harvesting and preparing medicinal herbs–can lower stress levels, and can also help support the immune system to help prevent or treat colds or infections.

Many people use herbal medicine to deal with insomnia (difficulty sleeping) and sleep problems such as sleep apnea due to a condition called obstructive sleep apnea (OSA). Because it is a sedative, valerian root can help to calm the nerves and improve sleep. Chamomile acts similarly in the body.

In addition, valerian root (used for sleep disorders) together with passionflower (used for anxiety disorders) can help with panic attacks. Some people use them to help with insomnia too.

History of Herbal Medicine

In the early history of every country across the globe, people lived in tribal societies. Many, if not all, tribal groups had some form of spiritual leader or medical practitioner, and in many societies, these two roles were combined. What is now called a 'shaman' was a person in each tribe that connected the spiritual world to the lives of the people, and often this included using plant medicine to heal wounds, illnesses, and other issues.

Notable groups in history were the Incas, Aztecs, Navajo, Cree, Slavic tribes, Germanic tribes, Celtic tribes, and Mongolian peoples. Of course, the 'shamanic' role has existed throughout every area of the world in the history of human society. We have always depended on nature and plant medicine to make sense of our illnesses and keep ourselves and our families healthy.

Traditions like herbalism, which have been passed down over generations, are a testament to how much more our predecessors understood the human body and health than we give them credit for. Although they couldn't explain it in scientific terms, there was a connection between the chemicals in plants and the needs of our bodies that our ancestors understood well.

Herbal medicine can be traced back 60,000 years and literature dating back to 1500 BCE has been found in Egypt, China, and India. All this folklore evolved over the centuries to become traditional medicine in different regions.

Plants are critical constituents of some of the most well-known and widely used medicines, which may surprise you. The medical world understands the power of plants, yet today, herbal medicine is often dismissed by doctors as a possible therapy. And this is primarily due to politics and the lack of understanding of modern medicine. But, many herbal remedies have been proven to be very effective in the healing process. And despite what some might say, medical records have shown that herbal medicine can be a vital part of our health.

Shamanism, a type of spirit medicine still practiced in many parts of the world, was used to learn about a plant's healing capabilities in many early societies. Some Shamans converse with plants (referred to as "plant teachers") to learn about other plants and healing practices.

There appears to be an intuitive relationship between humans and plants, allowing some sensitive people to tune in to the healing power of plants in specific situations. "Herbalists" is the term used to describe persons like this.

It is not uncommon for a herbalist to have a well-connected network with local health practitioners, natural foods stores, and farmers. A herbalist may be consulted as a consultation when issues arise or doctors diagnose problems.

Historical records of herbal remedies are some of the earliest accounts of treatments by human beings. Over 10,000 years ago, ancient Chinese herbalists created a book that contained 365 entries showing how to treat 365 diseases (modern herbalists call the book "The Tablets of the Lord of Tai Sui"). These herbs and remedies were used by Chinese doctors in 2,200 BCE.

Natural remedies like pure water have also been found to be effective on many occasions when used alongside modern medicine.

Plants are said to have been used to fight diseases since ancient times. In China, there was a picture of a plant that was planted in the tomb to help prevent people from dying there.

During the Middle Ages, herbalists that were seen as "witches" were burned at the stake in many towns. However, they were considered the only ones with the healing powers to deal with disease, and this is why many herbalists today still honor their healing powers.

Indeed, plants cannot speak, but they are not simple chemical compounds either. The properties of medicinal plants can vary greatly. Some species of plants can be found in the rainforest, ocean, or desert. Others grow in arctic regions and are used by those people to heal skin rashes or infections that occur during cold weather. All plants have some healing qualities and have been used for centuries for healing purposes by many cultures worldwide.

The ability of a plant to heal is essential to our very existence as humans. There are many plants from all over the world, and millions remain undiscovered by modern medicine.

Today, plants are used as integral ingredients in pharmaceuticals and used in food. It is also possible to create a new medicine from certain plant species, and our modern medicine relies on the unique chemical compounds found in plant remedies.

For example, the active ingredient of aspirin is acetylsalicylic acid, which is derived from the salicin found in willow bark. Exactly how aspirin works is currently unknown; however, it is suggested that the drug works by blocking the COX-1 and COX-2 enzymes in our body (COX-2 enzymes are linked with increased susceptibility to inflammatory diseases).

The active ingredients of many other drugs also come from plants.

Many plant remedies are also used as food. Some of the most common foods today have been used for their medicinal properties for centuries, such as ginger and garlic.

The political, economic, and scientific consequences of viewing plant medicines as merely chemical substances rather than dynamic spirits were significant. Many people began to revolt against these beliefs, but there was also an increase in chemicals.

The medical profession of that time generated much skepticism of herbal remedies, and many political leaders did not trust medicinal plants. Many countries made it illegal to be a herbalist.

This was not the only obstacle faced by herbalists in those days; they faced the opposition of their doctors and other physicians, who believed that plants were inferior and could never help heal suffering bodies.

In the 1990s, medicine began to take a more holistic approach, relying less on harsh drugs with potentially lethal side effects. This shift has rekindled interest in plant therapies, which have fewer side effects than pharmaceuticals. Herbal treatments are also less expensive than many prescription drugs.

Botanical medications were used 380% more in the United States between 1990 and 1997. According to Nutraceuticals World, by 2010, the global retail sale of botanical dietary supplements had surpassed $25 billion. In the coming decade, the dietary supplement market is predicted to grow and become one of the fastest-growing industries.

In addition to these benefits, herbal remedies are often more effective than pharmaceuticals, and they can be used with few side effects.

Myths And Facts About Herbal Medicines

Herbal medicine is riddled with myths and misconceptions. Some are somewhat true, but many deter individuals from trying a highly successful treatment method. Here's the truth regarding some of the most common urban legends.

1. Herbal Remedies Can Cure Anything.

Herbal treatments are effective in treating various diseases, but they have no curative properties. Garlic, for example, has long been misunderstood as a "wonder herb" that can treat just about anything, for example, cancers, AIDS, and even infertility.

However, that is not the case for many ailments that people believe are healed with garlic. Even though this notion is backed up by research, garlic has never been shown to be a cure for AIDS. It has been found to help slow the progression of the virus by inhibiting some of its functions and preventing it from spreading throughout cells. The myth is that it cures everything because it is a potent antibiotic, which is not true; garlic cannot heal anything, it can only help reduce the symptoms of an infection.

Herbal remedies should be used to complement conventional medicine, not as a substitute for pharmaceuticals. Using herbs as a substitute for pharmaceuticals can be very dangerous because the herbs may interact with each other, and toxic compounds from the herbs may interfere with medicines.

2. You Can Take too much of an Herbal Remedy.

Excessive use of herbs like ginseng, ginkgo, vitamin E, beta carotene, and many others can be toxic. Some herbs are to be used in extreme moderation. Formulas with more than 5% of the active ingredients should not be taken more than once a day because it is easy to take too much.

3. The FDA Does Not Regulate Herbs.

The FDA does not regulate herbal remedies since they are neither food nor drug. They simply restrict their use, sale, and distribution. Even though the FDA does not directly regulate herbs, that does not mean that there are no regulations regarding herbs at all. The FDA can take any product off the shelves if it contains an illegal ingredient. In other areas of the world, such as some European countries, food and drug associations do include herbal medicines in their regulations and therefore allow more legitimate and common use of herbal medicine in health care.

Herbal remedies are still chemicals, so take care and consideration while they are active in your system, especially if you are taking frequent and routine doses. All the same, warnings apply here as they do with prescription medicines such as those taken by heart patients and high blood pressure, blood clotting, and cholesterol patients.

4. Herbal Remedies Cannot Cure Cancer.

Many herbal medicines have been used to treat cancer and other disorders for hundreds of years. One such herb is Echinacea, which has been found to stimulate the immune system and may be effective in treating cancer cells. Some alternative cancer treatments include:

Arctium lappa (burdock root) and Taraxacum officinale (dandelion) are used in the treatment of breast, lymphatic, gastrointestinal, prostate, cervical, and lung cancer. The active ingredients in these herbicides are believed to have anti-cancer properties.

5. Herbal Medicine is Only Effective in Fighting Viral Infections.

Herbal medicine is extremely useful in treating viral diseases such as the common cold, flu, and contagious illnesses. It can also be used to treat bacterial infections such as strep throat, bacterial pneumonia, and meningitis.

6. Herbal Remedies Are Not Addictive.

One of the most common myths about herbs is that they are not addictive. However, some people can develop a psychological dependence on herbs when they take them daily. Herbs like St. John's Wort affect serotonin levels in the brain and can have adverse effects if taken continuously, so it is essential to consult a physician before taking them.

7. Herbal Medicines Don't Work The Same as Pharmaceuticals.

Some people believe that herbal medicines don't work as well as other forms of medicine. However, this is not strictly true. Herbal treatments have been used to cure a variety of disorders for ages, and they are equally effective as pharmaceuticals, according to studies. They work as well as pharmaceuticals and have many of the same kinds of side effects. In some instances, they can even be more effective than prescription medicines.

8. Herbal Medicine Is The Same As Homeopathy.

No, herbal medicine is not the same as homeopathy. Homeopathy requires that the remedy be diluted over and over again until it becomes so diluted that only a single molecule of the original substance remains. This is impossible to achieve with a pure herb.

9. It's Okay To Take Natural Medicines Along With Conventional Therapies.

Many people make the mistake of taking herbs along with their other medications. You must talk to your doctor before you add or eliminate anything from your daily treatment plan.

10. Herbal Medicine is Natural, so it's Always Safe.

Some individuals think herbs are "always safe" since they are natural. This is not true. Some herbs can be poisonous, so even though they come from plants, there is a chance of them containing toxic substances. This is why, before utilizing any herb as a therapeutic approach, you should always consult with a competent herbalist.

11. There's No Research About Herbal Medicine.

A lot of people depend on anecdotal evidence about herbal remedies and base their decisions about whether to try them on this information alone. In addition, there are a lot of unregulated forms of herbal medicine that are not verifiable. Books, journals, the internet, and experienced practitioners all provide a lot of information.

More than three-quarters of the population of poor countries use herbal medicine as their primary health care, according to estimates from the World Health Organization. Herbal medications and their ingredients provide long-term wellness benefits and can be utilized to cure human diseases and disorders effectively.

Herbs usually include a variety of active chemicals that might cause drug-like effects in the body. A significant range of herbs is effective in treating a variety of ailments. New technologies have been established to explore the biological significance of herbal medications in diverse human diseases and disorders as a result of recent breakthroughs in biology and medicine. As a result, it is critical to comprehend the mechanism(s) of action of herbal drugs to gain knowledge and design effective therapies.

Several fascinating papers outlining the efficacy of herbal medications in a variety of human diseases and disorders are included in this special edition.

The treatment of Si-Jun-Zi decoction, a well-known Chinese medicine, enhances the restoration of intestinal function after obstruction by controlling intestinal homeostasis. (Yang, L., et al, 2018).

TZQ-F has long been used in traditional Chinese medicine to treat diabetes. In healthy Chinese volunteers, H. Yuhong et al. examined the pharmacologic effects and gastrointestinal side events of TZQ-F and acarbose.

T. Numata et al. published a study that used the traditional Japanese herbal cure Saikokeishikankyoto to treat post-traumatic stress disorder (PTSD) in earthquake and tsunami survivors in Japan. Traditional medicine may be an effective treatment option for PTSD sufferers' psychological and physical symptoms.

We believe that readers and scientists working in the field of herbal pharmaceuticals will find not only an updated review of the subject in this book, but also a collection of accurate data on the efficacy of herbal drugs in a variety of lifestyle diseases and disorders, together with their proposed mechanisms of action.

How to Maximize the Benefits of Herbal Medicine Safely?

Herbal medicines should not be used to cure a serious illness; instead, they should be used as a supplement to other treatments. When taking herbs, always seek medical guidance.

If you don't know how much is too much when using herbs, leave it at the first sign of an adverse effect, for instance, nausea and vomiting, because this is a sign that your body doesn't tolerate the herb well at all.

Incorporate herbal remedies with water, tea, food, milk, or smoothies.

Do not take herbal remedies if you experience heart palpitations or have unexplained fainting spells. Many people who have taken herbs experience extreme anxiety while they are taking the remedy, which can be life-threatening in some cases.

Any packaged herbal product in stores will have warnings on the label. Make sure, if you are pregnant, to check that it is safe to consume during pregnancy. It is not always the case that natural products are safe for mothers and unborn babies.

Use herbs as a complementary treatment instead of relying on them entirely. Always consult with your physician concerning what herbs to take and how to take them.

Don't offer children herbal treatments without first visiting a doctor. Children are particularly susceptible to the bad effects of herbs, so make sure that any plant you give them does not cause them any harm.

Herbal remedies can be extremely effective but must be used properly and safely for maximum effectiveness.

Despite these myths, herbal medicine and the use of plants in medicine are becoming more popular in the West. Many individuals are increasingly aware that, rather than relying entirely on conventional treatments, it is preferable to take care of the body through dietary and lifestyle adjustments.

With this awareness comes a new interest in herbalism, which has given birth to new fields such as ethnopharmacology, ethnobotany, and phytochemistry. This allows individuals to test the efficacy of plants that have been in use for a long time. Many believe that there is so much untapped potential in herbal medicine, and they see this new field as a way to make herbs more accessible to common people. However, many skeptics worry about health risks and the ethics around using wild plants as medicine on a wider scale.

Ethnobotany refers to the study of plant medicines used by indigenous peoples in traditional societies.

Plants were the primary source of medicines before advances in synthetic chemistry and the discovery of antimicrobials in the late 19th and early 20th centuries. For centuries, medicine was based solely on plant-based treatments. More than 95% of conventional drugs and vaccines before the 20th century were based on plant extracts. Many of these traditional medicines are still in use today and are known as ethnobotanical drugs or ethnomedicines.

Foreign pharmaceuticals designed to mimic the effects of nature's own medicines (e.g., ginseng) have also been used in some traditional medicines to preserve their effect during long journeys, pharmacological isolation, and storage.

Plant-derived therapeutic medicines account for more than 20% of the ethical turnover of pharmaceutical companies today. More than 7 million people in the United States alone are using over-the-counter and prescription herbal medications to improve their health.

The worldwide market for herbal medicines is estimated at around $12 billion per year (Gwynn, J., & Hylands, P. 2022).

In recent years, the usage of herbal therapeutic goods and supplements has increased, but so has the risk of injury. Adverse effects of these products are frequently overlooked.

Moreover, current international guidelines and regulatory standards for herbal medicines differ among countries and regions, making harmonized global safety monitoring of these substances challenging.

This post discusses the challenges related to adverse reactions from herbal medicinal products and supplements and provides suggestions on how best to address these challenges. We also offer a primer on regulatory frameworks for herbal medicines in different regions of the world.

The Global Status of Herbal Medicinal Products and their Regulation

Today, herbal medicinal products are used by more than half of the population in developed countries and by 10-15%

of the world's population. In some Asian countries, where herbs remain a dominant form of primary health care and usage is growing in many other regions, including Africa and Latin America, herbal medicines have become an essential part of health care. They are available as foods and dietary supplements, traditional medicines (in pharmacies or by practitioners), and prescribed medications (by physicians).

The popularity of herbal medicines is largely attributable to the perception that they are "natural," safe, and effective. In addition, they are often used as a first-line therapy or as an adjunct to conventional medications.

Herbal medicinal products are marketed in capsules, tablets, creams, teas, or tinctures. Tinctures—where extracts from herbs are dissolved in alcohol and taken orally –are generally derived from the fresh whole plant. In this case, herbal medicines are referred to as "botanical medicines." In many countries, the safety and quality of herbal medicines are not regulated. Regulation of these items is well developed in several countries, such as the United States, Canada, Japan, and Australia. However, the regulatory frameworks in place in these countries have limitations regarding enforceability and oversight.

In some regions of the world (including South America), herbs may be regulated as foods and therefore fall under the domain of food safety authorities or health departments.

Several factors have been ascribed to the current rise of popular interest in herbal medicines, including:

- Increased awareness (and the perception) that these drugs are safer than conventional medicines.

- Promotion by practitioners of alternative medicine, who often combine herbal and other medicine with conventional treatments.

- The growth of global consumerism has led to greater self-medication and greater use of alternative therapies as an option for healthcare.

- Various new consumer markets in developed countries, including baby boomers looking to replace their pharmaceuticals with botanical supplements.

- Consumers can now perform their own research, gather information, and compare shops, thanks to the growth of the internet.

- The use of herbal medicines in traditional medicine practices in developed countries.

- Due to the widespread availability of herbal products in local markets and pharmacies, many people who are not regular users purchase these products for self-medication.

- Government policy and regulation, which has led to the development of national and regional regulatory frameworks in some countries.

Aside from the aforementioned factors, there are a few more to think about. Numerous herbal medicine producers' and sales representatives' marketing techniques and efforts have helped to bring these products into the spotlight. In particular, herbal medicine makers frequently claim that their products are safe or very useful for a variety of disorders and ailments.

Product regulations (including good manufacturing practices, good laboratory practices, good consumer protection, and hazard communication) are used to ensure product quality, safety, and efficacy.

Regulation of herbal medicinal products varies among countries and regions. Some countries have specific policies for herbal medicinal products; others use generic regulatory guidelines.

It is known that public misperceptions and awareness are a major influence on the use of herbal medicinal products. To effectively prevent adverse reactions, it is important to know what consumers believe about these products. In addition, one must understand how changes in policy or regulation may affect consumers' perception of the benefits and risks of herbal medicinal products.

Since 1998, the European Union's Food and Drug Freedom of System (FFS) policy has mandated that the European Commission monitor and report on consumer perceptions of herbal medicines. This is because the lack of quality assurance, standardization, and regulation in the manufacturing and distribution process has contributed to the misperception that herbal remedies are perfectly safe.

The FFS was strengthened in 2005 with a focus on herbal medicinal products and consumer attitudes to safety, efficacy, and quality. In particular, the FFS survey aimed to evaluate consumer attitudes towards or knowledge of herbal medicinal products in several countries. It also aimed to provide evidence of consumers' willingness to use herbal medicines as part of their primary health care.

Herbal medicines should be considered with caution because some plants contain toxic substances and/or natural chemical compounds that can result in adverse health effects. As with all medications, the potential for adverse reactions is enhanced by the use of other substances that might interact with their use. Caution, and knowing what a plant may contain is necessary when practicing herbal medicine.

This report evaluates each of the 74 herbal medicinal products in this review, focusing on factors that could affect their safety and efficacy. Other sections of this report include a general description of herbal medicine, an overview of its primary manufacturing processes, and an assessment of available data on safety and efficacy (Ekor, 2022).

CHAPTER TWO:
STEP 1 - HAVE A GOOD GRASP OF
HERBS

Every good mind starts somewhere, and when it comes to herbs, a new journey should always start with getting the appropriate knowledge. This knowledge will be your guide when you're creating your remedies.

In this chapter, you will learn about the letter H in our herbal medicine HEALING framework, meaning "have a good grasp of herbs." You will learn the various types of herbs, what they are used for, and some of the ways that they are used.

Conventional vs. Herbal Medicine

Conventional medicine refers to modern medical practice and to its method of prevention, diagnosis, and treatment of disease. 'Conventional' medicine is usually preferred by those who are confident in its efficacy. This method is adopted by the western world, especially in North America and Europe. The medications used are pharmaceuticals and are made to address your symptoms, not cure the underlying cause of your disease—opposite from the intent of herbal medicine.

Herbal medicine is a subset of alternative medicine, and it is also commonly referred to as "natural" or "botanical" medicine. This type of medicine uses natural substances found in plants— herbs, fruits, and vegetables. Because this method is holistic, it treats the root cause of the complaint rather than just masking symptoms. It is most often used for treating minor ailments, and it takes a little longer to reach its effects in comparison to your conventional drug. However, natural remedies may not require a prescription and can be more easily accessible.

Simply put, pharmaceuticals are a temporary fix for a problem, whereas natural medicines restore function and last a lifetime.

As shocking as it may sound, pharmaceutical drugs result in more deaths compared to herbal medicines. Conventional medicines are highly regulated by the government, and so manufacturers are obliged to report even suspected adverse drug reactions. In the United States of America, about 8% of hospital admissions are due to adverse or side effects of synthetic medications (Ali Karimi, 2022).

Conventional medicines can be toxic to you in the long run. Approximately 100,000 people each year die due to these toxicities. This is not saying that herbal medicines are safer, but the fact is there are fewer complications compared to conventional medications. Herbal medicine also has fewer side effects, and long-term use of these products can improve your health rather than cause it to deteriorate.

Moreover, drug residues may linger in the body even after the drug has left the system. This can result in various disorders, some of which can be life-threatening.

Two people in San Francisco ended up in intensive care after trying herbal therapy. The incident is expected to raise questions about the safety of herbal medicine. Are they, on the other hand, any more harmful than medicines from your doctor or those purchased without a prescription over the counter?

Herbal remedies are considered safer than your conventional medication. Because they are natural products, they do not have the same level of toxicity as your conventional medications. However, it is best to be aware of possible allergic reactions to herbal remedies. Herbal medicines should not be used for treating serious or life-threatening illnesses unless you have consulted a health professional or physician beforehand (Booker, 2022).

Herbal remedies can also be harmful if you ignore the 'side effects.' Although less severe, some side effects can occur, such as nausea and vomiting. Always consult your pharmacist or doctor when you're in doubt.

If you are taking conventional medications, it does not mean that you should stop taking them. Rather you should consult a physician or your pharmacist before trying herbal remedies since not all of them may be safe for use in combination with conventional medications.

Herbal medicine is preferred for treating non-life-threatening conditions and minor ailments because it is more holistic, has broader complementary or synergistic actions on the body, rarely has adverse effects, is considered long-lasting, and helps restore function, whereas conventional medicines are targeted toward specific symptoms.

Why Should You Pick Herbal Remedies?

Herbal medicines should be considered if you are a supporter of alternative medicine. Although both types of medication are designed to help promote your health and alleviate pain and other symptoms of illnesses, they do so in different ways. Some of the advantages of using herbal treatments rather than drugs are listed below.

1. Herbal medicines work.

If you prefer alternative therapy to conventional treatment, herbal remedies are the way to go. Herbal medicines are natural and do not have a lot of side effects, and they work. In some cases, conventional medicines do not work as well as herbal remedies. Every minute counts when you are sick, and herbal remedies can work fast and be on-hand when you need them.

2. Herbal medicines tend to be safer than pharmaceuticals.

Pharmaceutical manufacturing is a chemical-heavy process. These chemicals are then processed and added to the product. In the end, a lot of harmful substances are created and might cause health issues later down the road. Natural herbal remedies are made from natural products such as plants, fruits, or vegetables. It's mind-boggling to think that a plant can have all these natural attributes and be safe to use. Modern medicine has been able to extract and create synthetic drugs, but herbal remedies are free from preservatives and other chemicals that cause many side effects.

3. Herbal medicines are usually a less expensive choice.

Most herbal remedies are relatively affordable. You do not have to splurge on your medication, and you can afford natural treatment. It's a pleasant thing knowing that you are not hurting yourself and the environment just because of the medication you choose to take. As we continue to see selfish corporate pharmaceutical executives drive up the price of their products, it's reassuring to know that natural options are often less expensive than their pharmaceutical counterparts.

4. Herbal medicine is the pinnacle of long-term health.

Herbal remedies are the best therapy approach to better health. That's because herbals do not simply suppress symptoms; they work to correct the underlying issue. Although healing herbs have been used for thousands of years, we are still learning more about their power.

Herbal medicines can promote wellness without causing addiction and the most common side effects of herbal remedies are usually negligible or harmless. The biggest concern is that you might experience some mild allergic reaction when taking herbal medicine. If you feel the reaction, stop using it and see a doctor immediately

5. Herbal medicines and pharmaceuticals may interact.

They are, after all, both drugs. They both contain chemical compounds, but they are not the same. The main difference is that herbs usually contain very few side effects, while pharmaceuticals may cause a multitude of side effects. Some natural supplements can interact with prescription medications. By taking the two together, you are putting your health at risk. As a result, before taking both, see your doctor or a certified herbalist.

6. Always make sure you're using the correct part of the plant.

Some plant parts aren't good for humans. You should not use herbal remedies on just anyone's advice but instead, see a professional. Do your research on herbs and botanicals that are safe to use for your condition — and always, always follow the directions on the label.

Using the wrong plant portion may affect how effective your remedy is. This can be dangerous. However, make sure to always use the correct part of the plant when creating your remedy.

One of the most important things you need to know about herbal remedies is what type of herb you are using as a "herb core" for your remedy. Once you know what type of herb is used in an herbal remedy, you'll know how to use it in your healing remedy and when it's suitable for how you want to use it.

Herbs are categorized by their parts—roots, stems, leaves, flowers, and fruits. Each part of the plant gives a unique benefit you can use to treat a specific ailment. Often people toss the different parts of plants and forget about them in their remedies. This is very dangerous because you could be tossing the most potent parts of each herb in your remedy.

7. Most herbs have dozens, if not hundreds, of different therapeutic components.

The components of the phytochemicals in plants are complex and can include hundreds of therapeutic properties. These healing compounds naturally occur in herbs, and herbal remedies can help to treat a multitude of ailments, or multiple symptoms at one time. Each plant could be a remedy for several ailments.

8. Herbs should not be treated in the same manner that pharmaceuticals are.

Herbs work on a holistic level, and the way they heal is not the same as the way drugs do. Herbs help to promote overall health and wellbeing, but they should never be used in place of pharmaceuticals.

Pharmaceutical drugs targeted toward specific symptoms elicit a specific reaction, with side effects considered normal and expected. Herbs contain healing compounds that work on the body more holistically, rather than targeting one specific symptom, which is why herbs are considered to be complementary and are used in conjunction with conventional medications.

Misidentification of herbs can lead to severe side effects. You may be searching for a plant in the wild, but instead find its similar-looking plant. This can be a problem, as you do not know the real constituents in the plant you have found, and they could be ineffective for you, or toxic.

You will never be prescribed or sold a poisonous plant by a professional, but you may be advised to use a remedy that is not effective for you. Talk with your practitioner if a remedy causes any adverse reaction, such as an allergy, or if it seems ineffective, and another remedy will be chosen.

Be sure you know exactly what you need and the weeds that should be eliminated in your yard before you even think of picking up your herbal remedy.

An example is the Western US 'death camas' plant. It is often mistaken for the edible wild onion, but is very toxic. We will lay out some tips for identifying plants in the wild below

In an age of global warming, it's good to know that there are natural remedies out there that can help us survive. Herbs are the most powerful and versatile tools that an individual can have. Some herbs can be turned into essential oils, and others can be used to heal wounds, while some are good for relieving headaches.

This book will assist you in becoming familiar with a variety of medicinal herbs, as well as their purposes, abilities, and effects in the promotion of health and healing.

There are a lot of different herbals, and you need to be able to identify which herbs are supposed to be used for what. Knowing these things will help you in your herbal journey.

Let's get started, shall we?

Echinacea

Other Names:

- Black Sampson

- Black Sampson Echinacea

- Narrow-Leaf Coneflower

Scientific Name: *Echinacea purpurea*

About Echinacea:

A flowering plant, part of the larger daisy family (Asteraceae), petals may be pink or purple, surrounding a seed head that is spiky and dark brown or red. Native Americans loved this plant, and it was used for numerous ailments like colds, infections, and many others. Today, many companies have taken hold of the echinacea and have turned it into over-the-counter herbs for the flu and the common cold.

The upper section and the echinacea roots are useful for herbal supplements, and they are even extracted and used in teas, tablets, and tinctures. Antioxidants like Rosmarinic acid are abundant in it. Flavonoids and Cichoric acid help the immune system fight oxidative stress.

Used for:

- Wounds

- Burns

- Toothaches

- Sore throat

- Reducing the risk of colds

Other benefits:

- Reduces inflammation

- Improves immunity

- Lowers blood sugar levels

Medicinal Parts:

- Leaves

- Petals

- Roots (many believe roots have the strongest effect)

Consumed by: Taken as tea or supplement, but also applied topically

Possible side effects: nausea, stomach pain, and skin rash have occasionally been reported

Other important notes: 3 types of Echinacea are used for herbal remedies

- E. angustifolia, which has narrow petals

- E. pallida, which has pale petals

- E. purpurea, which has purple petals

Ginseng

Other Names: Quinquefolius

Scientific Name: *Panax ginseng*

About Ginseng:

An Araliaceae family plant that is native to the deciduous forests of the Appalachian and Ozark regions of North America. The root of this plant is extremely valuable in medicine. Only the most skilled spiritual leaders use it in medicine. This root can be used to treat digestive issues and relieve pain.

Used For:

- Erectile dysfunction

- High blood sugar

- Stress

- Inflammation

- Flu

- Memory loss

- Issues with digestion

- Sleeping disorders

Other Benefits: It boosts metabolism in the body. It improves sexual performance, learning, and memory.

Medicinal Parts:

- Roots, especially dried

Consumed By: taken as a tea or dried to make powder

Possible Side Effects:

- If you have any hormone-related disorders, it is best to refrain from using ginseng as it can cause these conditions to worsen.

- Ginseng is not safe to use if you are pregnant. Ginseng has been linked to birth defects.

- If you are diabetic, consult a herbalist before using ginseng.

- Taking doses that are higher than what your herbalist recommends can lead to restlessness/insomnia.

- Some mental illnesses can be irritated by ginseng. This can lead to outbursts, frustration, and the inability to fall asleep.

Ginkgo

Other Names: ginkgo or ginkgo

Scientific Name: *Ginkgo biloba*

About Ginkgo:

Ginkgo biloba is a large, slow-growing perennial shrub that can live in an ancient wild era. The sole survivor of the oldest known genus of trees, Ginkgo is a medicinal plant native to the northern hemisphere. This herb is used not only for its flavor but for its medicinal properties.

Used For:

- Heart disease

- Dementia

- Mental difficulties

- Sexual dysfunction.

Other Benefits:

- Ginkgo improves memory in people with Alzheimer's disease, dementia, and other brain diseases.

- Aids memory and improves other brain-related health conditions.

- Helps with psychological problems such as depression and ADHD

- Ginkgo also improves alertness, which is vital for exercise and sports. It increases energy, so it is recommended for athletes.

Medicinal Parts:

- Seeds

- Leaves

Consumed By:

The seeds and leaves are traditionally used to prepare teas and tinctures, although leaf extract is employed in most modern applications.

Possible Side Effects:

- Headache

- Heart palpitations

- Digestive issues

- Skin reactions

- Increased risk of bleeding

Elderberry

Other Names: Elder, Sambucus

Scientific Name: *Sambucus nigra*

About Elderberry:

This bushy shrub can grow up to 33 feet. The stems that emerge from the ground have dark brown bark, often with vertical fissures. The opposite leaves are composite, oval-shaped with a pointed tip, bright green, with serrated margins, and hairy at the leafstalk and base. The white (or cream, depending on the species) flowers are arranged in large clusters at the top of the plant. Fruits are round berries whose color may vary from one species to another: red for Sambucus racemosa, blue for Sambucus cerulea, and almost black for nigra.

The leaves are oppositely arranged. Each leaf is 5 to 30 cm long. The color of the flowers ranges from white to cream. Belongs to the Adoxaceae family.

Used For:

- High cholesterol

- Colds

- Influenza

- CFS or chronic fatigue syndrome

- Constipation

- Obesity

- Headaches

- Gingivitis

- Swine flu

- Tooth pain

Other Benefits:

- And can even help prevent heart disease

Medicinal Parts:

- The roots

- Inner bark

- Leaves

- Berries

Consumed By:

An infusion, associated, if you want, with violet and thyme for respiratory conditions or in elderberry syrup. And the infusion alone or combined with plantain to treat bedwetting. An alternative is the application of cold compresses, soaked with this infusion, on the back, which will calm the impulses of the bladder.

Possible Side Effects:

Excessive consumption of berries can cause poisoning.

Other Important Notes:

Elderberry (fruit) may be dried in a food dryer, then frozen and used in cooking throughout the cold months for disease prevention. Flowers may be gathered in June, dried, and made into tea. Before eating the flowers, cut away the stems and remove the stems from the berries as well.

St. John's Wort

Other Names:

- Amber

- Barbe de Saint-Jean

- Chasse-diable

- Demon Chaser

- Fuga Daemonum

- Goatweed, Hardha

Scientific Name: *Hypericum perforatum*

About St. John's Wort:

An upright, woody herb that grows in temperate areas. It was traditionally believed to ward off evil on St. John's feast and hence got its name.

Used For:

- Wound healing

- Alleviate insomnia

- Depression

- Kidney diseases

- Lung diseases

- Moderate depression.

Other Benefits:

- Helpful in treating mood disorders

Medicinal Parts:

- Flower

Consumed By:

- Used to make teas

- Capsules

- Extracts

Possible Side Effects:

- Allergic reactions

- Dizziness

- Confusion

- Dry mouth

- Increased light sensitivity

Turmeric

Other Names: Curcumin

Scientific Name: *Curcuma longa*

About Turmeric:

Turmeric is commonly found in kitchens, especially in Indian or other south-east Asian homes. The root or rhizome of curcuma longa is so potent, it is used for some of the most powerful inflammation and cancer-preventing remedies available. The fresh root is best, but mostly you will see the dried powdered root in stores.

Used For:

- Weight gain

- Aid in weight loss

- Inflammation

- Swelling

- Pain

- Metabolic syndromes

- Anxiety

Other Benefits:

Turmeric can be consumed either in a pill or powder form. Add turmeric powder to your everyday recipes to reap the health benefits of turmeric.

Medicinal Parts:

- Root

Consumed By:

- Used as a spice in several dishes, or pressed into capsules, or made into smoothies and milk drinks.

Possible Side Effects:

High doses may lead to:

- Diarrhea

- Headache

- Skin irritation

Ginger

Other Names: Ginger root

Scientific Name: *Zingiber officinale*

About Ginger:

Ginger is a yellow root with brown-colored skin. Many have been using it for years as a spice or flavoring on their plate of food or drink. It's been used to treat digestive problems, indigestion, nausea, and a range of ailments for centuries.

Used For:

- Treats nausea

- Indigestion

- Reduces inflammation

- Improves circulation

- Clears sinuses and congestion.

Other Benefits:

- Native Americans used this herb for dysentery and chills.

- The Chinese use it for nausea and other digestive ailments.

- It is also a natural diuretic and mild blood thinner that lowers blood pressure.

- Ginger is used in the treatment of pain relief from headaches, toothaches, sore throats, backaches, cold sores, and many forms of cancer like colon cancer.

Medicinal Parts:

- Root

Consumed By:

Taken as tea or tincture, used as a spice in cooking, or even grated into food or drinks.

Possible Side Effects:

Stomach pain or bloating has been reported in some people, especially those who take large doses or are new to the plant.

Other Important Notes:

Ginger is not recommended for pregnant women. It might cause uterine contractions if consumed in excess.

Valerian

Other Names: Wild Valerian

Scientific Name: *Valeriana officinalis*

About Valerian:

Valerian is a 3-foot-tall perennial plant. The flowers are small, pink with five petals. The stem is stout, and the leaves are long and narrow. In most countries, the root of valerian is used in some form or another. The roots of this plant have a very distinct and strong odor.

Used For:

- Natural remedy to help with insomnia

- Anxiety

- Stress-related problems

Other Benefits:

- Valerian root can also be used as a sedative and muscle relaxer.

Medicinal Parts:

- Roots

- Leaves

Consumed By:

- It is available in several forms, including tea, tincture, and capsules.

Possible Side Effects:

- This plant should not be consumed by people who have high blood pressure.

- Diabetics should stay away from taking it because it may reduce glucose tolerance.

- It may also cause nausea and headache and make you feel groggy.

- Some have reported sleepiness and/or drowsiness as a side effect of using valerian.

Other Important Notes:

Valerian should not be used long term for treating insomnia. Some rare side effects should be kept in mind. Teas made from this plant can cause heart problems (heartbeat may be accelerated) or even stop it completely if too much is taken. It may also make you dizzy and confused. This herb may also cause weight gain, especially if you take too much of the herb over a long period.

Chamomile

Other Names: Common Chamomile

Scientific Name: *Matricaria chamomilla*

About Chamomile:

The daisy-like flowers are blue, white, or pink. The plant grows all over the United States but is most common in the Midwest and Northeast. It is also found in the warmer areas of Canada and Mexico. Chamomile has been used for well over 3,000 years in the East. The plant is often grown for its flowers, which are beautiful and make an excellent addition to a flower garden. The plant itself is hardy but must be grown in a sunny location to grow well. Chamomile blooms are easily recognized by their small, yellow flowers with long stamens. The leaves are narrow, have saw-edges, and have an aroma similar to apples.

Used For:

- Antiseptic

- Antibacterial

- Chamomile can be used to reduce swelling and pain.

Other Benefits:

- Chamomile is used as a natural remedy for digestive disorders, colic in babies, diarrhea, gas, and bloating.

- It is also used to treat skin inflammation and infections.

- If you have a cold or flu, you can use chamomile to help reduce the symptoms of it.

- It has been proven that chamomile can kill bacteria like MRSA that cause infections.

- You can even drink the tea for coughs and sore throats.

- The flowers and leaves are both used as tea to help promote healthy digestion.

Medicinal Parts:

- Leaves

- Flowers

- Stems

Consumed By:

- Taken as a tea or tincture.

Possible Side Effects:

- Many people are allergic to plants in the Asteraceae family, to which Chamomile belongs.

- Chamomile *is* recommended for pregnant women because it helps with nausea, heartburn, gas, and bloating. It also helps relieve stress.

Other Important Notes:

The one caveat to using chamomile is that it can function as a sedative in big doses. So be careful not to overdo it.

Feverfew

Other Names: Altamisa

Scientific Name: Tanacetum parthenium

About Feverfew:

The flowers are small, yellow, and white with five petals. The plant can be found in most sections of the United States, and it grows up to three feet tall. In some areas, the flowers bloom all year. The leaves are tiny, thin, lance-shaped, and serrated on the margins. The blooms are delicious as well and can be eaten raw.

Used For:

- Used to relieve muscle and joint pain, especially in women.

- Fever reduction

- Inflammation

- Neuralgia (nerve pain)

- Rheumatoid arthritis

- Menstrual disorders.

Other Benefits:

- Native Americans produced tea from feverfew roots that are said to help relieve symptoms of depression.

Medicinal Parts:

- Leaves

- Flowers

- Roots

- Stems (the above-ground parts)

Consumed By:

- Taken as a tea or tincture

Possible Side Effects:

- None.

- Feverfew is recommended for pregnant women because it has been used to relieve morning sickness and headaches, as well as treat insomnia.

- Feverfew is also safe for children.

Other Important Notes:

Feverfew can cause blood clotting to slow down, so if you're taking any prescription medications, talk to your doctor before taking them.

Garlic

Other Names: Ail Blanc, Ail Cultivate

Scientific Name: *Allium sativum*

About Garlic:

Used For:

- Antibiotic

- Antifungal,

- Antiviral

- Antiparasitic

- Antimicrobial

Other Benefits:

- Cancer-fighting.

Medicinal Parts:

- Cloves

- Bulbs

Consumed By:

It is taken as a tea, crushed and mixed with water or oil, or even made into capsules. It can also be cooked, baked into bread, brewed into beer, or even eaten raw.

The medicinal effects are only activated when garlic is crushed or chopped up.

Possible Side Effects:

- It is not recommended for people with high blood pressure since it can raise blood pressure and increase the risk of heart disease.

- Abdominal pain

- Bad breath

- Nausea or bloating.

Other Important Notes:

Garlic is recommended for pregnant women because it can help with morning sickness and prevent bacterial infections. It is also safe to use during breastfeeding. Even though garlic has been used for hundreds of years - it can still have very strong side effects and should be taken with caution.

Milk Thistle

Other Names: Holy thistle

Scientific Name: *Carduus Marianus*

The white or yellow flowers are often purple at the base. The plant grows up to 2 feet tall and is found in most parts of the United States. The flower heads are also edible and can be used to make traditional flour. About Milk Thistle:

Used For:

- It has been used to treat stomach ulcers and liver disease.

- Milk Thistle is often taken to treat the bad effects of alcohol and prescription medications on the liver.

Other Benefits:

- It can also be used to strengthen the liver as a tonic.

Medicinal Parts:

- Leaves

- Flowers

Consumed By:

- Taken as a tea or tincture

Possible Side Effects:

- None.

- Milk Thistle is recommended for pregnant women because it has been used to reduce the symptoms of morning sickness and for those who are experiencing heavy bleeding during their menstrual cycle.

Other Important Notes:

Milk Thistle should not be used for more than six weeks at a time because it has been linked to abnormal cardiac function.

Saw Palmetto

Other Names: American Dwarf Palm Tree

Scientific Name: *Serenoa Repens*

About Saw Palmetto:

A flowering perennial wetland small tree or palm that generally grows as horizontal creepers and, more rarely, as erect trees.

The stems are fibrous rather than woody and typically grow below the surface. The leaves protrude above ground as large fan-shapes with long, thick, and sturdy petioles covered in saw-like teeth on either side. The leaves are like a palm tree, with several long and thin leaflets joining at the base in a zig-zag, folded pattern.

Several flowers grow on long stalks or panicles from the axils of the leaf. They are very small and yellow-white in color with no petals but modified, petal-like stamens leading to yellow tips. The flowers are highly attractive to bees. The fruits develop as fleshy, green, oval drupes that turn black when ripe.

Used For:

- Treatment of enlarged prostate glands in men.

- Treatment of acne

- Improving urinary function

Other Benefits:

- It has been used to treat irregular menstrual cycles and certain types of breast cancer in women.

Medicinal Parts:

- The leaves

Consumed By:

- Taken as a capsule or tea

Possible Side Effects:

- None when it is taken under medical supervision.

- Side effects may include mild stomach pain, gas, loose stools, or headaches.

Other Important Notes:

Saw Palmetto should not be used for more than six weeks at a time because it can cause problems with your heart and urinary tract. It is also not advised for children or women who are pregnant.

Calendula

Other Names: Marigold

Scientific Name: *Calendula officinalis*

About Calendula:

A small herb that can grow up to 3 feet in height, with bright yellow-to-orange flowers and a reddish-purple calyx. Calendula is a biennial plant that starts as a rosette of usually dark green leaves. These are covered with short, soft hairs and light dots along their edges known as stomata that help the plant breathe.

When the plant reaches full maturity, it will form long seed pods filled with small translucent seeds that are coated in a clear mucus that protects them from being eaten by certain insects. The seeds are also covered with a sticky coating and adhere to the fur or clothing of animals that eat them.

Used For:

- Used to treat burns and sunburns.

- Used as a soothing ointment for minor skin injuries and irritations.

- Used in many cosmetic creams to reduce wrinkles and smooth the surface of the skin.

- Used as a mild blood purifier.

- Used to treat stomach ulcers and the common cold.

Other Benefits:

- Help to get rid of warts and soothe the discomfort associated with hemorrhoids.

Medicinal Parts:

- The leaves

- Stems

- Flowers

Consumed By:

- It is usually taken in capsule form or as an infusion from the leaves.

- It can also be available in a cream, tincture, or ointment.

Possible Side Effects:

- None

Other Important Notes:

This herb is generally well tolerated by humans. However, it is possible for people that are allergic to plants in the daisy family—such as Ragweed—to have a bad reaction when consuming Calendula. If consuming Calendula regularly, it is best to limit the intake of high-fiber foods and avoid consuming alcohol or other stimulants.

Cilantro

Other Names: Coriander, Chinese Parsley

Scientific Name: *Coriandrum sativum*

About Cilantro:

The cilantro plant can grow anywhere from 1 to 3 feet tall and has green stems with dark green leaves. The leaves are broadly pinnate with three to five soft and smooth ovate (oval-shaped) and serrated leaflets.

Used For:

- Blood detoxifier

- Reduce anxiety, increase sleep quality

- It can be used as a spice or seasoning.

Other Benefits:

- It has powerful digestive characteristics and protects against heart disease and urinary problems.

- Cilantro is a diuretic, which means it can help to rid the body of toxins and excess fluids that are found in the bloodstream.

- It is also a natural astringent, which means it can help to shrink swollen or runny bladders by constricting or closing the bladder muscles.

- It can also help expel products of digestion with the help of its pressure-reducing properties.

Medicinal Parts:

- Leaves

- Stems

- Flowers

Consumed By:

- It is usually taken in capsule form or as an infusion from the leaves.

- Cilantro can also be available in a cream, tincture, or ointment

- Most commonly eaten fresh in meals.

Possible Side Effects:

- None

Lemon Balm

Other Names: Melissa

Scientific Name: *Melissa officinalis*

About Lemon Balm:

Used to treat:

- Digestive issues

- Repelling insects

- Minor pain relief

- Treating irritability

- Healthy brain function

Other Benefits:

- It can reduce swelling, inflammation, and pain. Lemon balm is also helpful in treating depression, anxiety, and migraines as well as helping to balance mood swings.

- Lemon balm has a relaxing impact on the nervous system, making it an efficient stress reliever.

Medicinal Parts:

- The leaves

- Stems

- Flowers

Consumed By:

- Usually taken in capsule form or as an infusion from the leaves. It is also available in a cream, tincture, or ointment.

Possible Side Effects:

- Lemon balm can alter thyroid performance. If you have any thyroid disorders, lemon balm might not be the best medicinal herb for your needs.

- Lemon balm can affect blood sugar levels; avoid the use or use with caution if you are diabetic.

Other Important Notes:

Pregnant or nursing women should keep away from lemon balm just as a precaution. While there have been no reported incidents with this herb concerning pregnancy or nursing an infant, there is just not enough viable research to confirm its safety when used during these times.

Peppermint

Other Names: Brandy Mint

Scientific Name: *Mentha piperita*

About Peppermint:

Peppermint is a small herb with many small, pointed leaves. The leaf stem is a narrow stalk that tapers off into several branches.

Used to treat:

- Cough and sore throats

- Headaches and migraines

- Diarrhea and nausea

Other Benefits:

- Peppermint is said to relieve cold symptoms such as a sore throat, cough, and congestion.

- In addition, it's also used for headaches, migraines, muscle aches, and cramps.

Medicinal Parts:

- Leaves

- Stems

- Seeds

Consumed By:

- Usually used as tea or taken in capsule form.

Possible Side Effects:

- The main side effect of peppermint is that it can cause stomach upset when taken in large amounts or with certain types of medication.

Other Important Notes:

Pregnant or nursing women should stay away from peppermint as this herb can cause stomach upsets. The effects of peppermint are believed to be passed through breast milk.

A 15-minute-long topical herbal steam bath has been recommended as a treatment for seasonal affective disorder.

Rosemary

Other Names: Compass Plant

Scientific Name: *Salvia rosmarinus*

About Rosemary:

Rosemary is a small evergreen shrub that grows in both arid and humid regions of the world. It produces small pink or white flowers arranged in dense panicles that are about 1.5-2.5cm long.

Used For:

- Digestive troubles

- Inflammation

- Teeth and gums

- Flatulence

- Bronchitis and asthma

- Minor pain relief.

- Healthy brain function.

Other Benefits:

- It is believed that rosemary has an invigorating effect on the brain, helping to ease depression and anxiety as well as aid concentration and memory.

- It is also used as an antioxidant and is thought to be a blood thinner.

- For generations, rosemary has been used to treat digestive problems such as gas and bloating, diarrhea, nausea, and indigestion.

- The essential oil of rosemary can help to ease the symptoms of minor aches, pains, and joint stiffness.

- It is also said to improve circulation while reducing the lactic acid build-up in the muscles. Rosemary is also said to lower cholesterol levels.

- Possible side effects:

- Rosemary can cause allergic reactions, especially in people with sensitive skin.

Medicinal Parts:

- The leaves

- Flowers

- Fruits

Consumed By:

- Usually used in tea form or as an infusion from the leaves and flowers.

- It is also available in tinctures, capsules, and essential oils.

Possible Side Effects:

- Rosemary can cause allergic reactions, especially in people with sensitive skin.

Other Important Notes:

When rosemary is eaten for medical purposes by humans, there are no documented harmful side effects. When applied to the skin, however, rosemary has been known to cause skin irritation or sensitization in a few cases.

Rosemary is not recommended for children and pregnant or nursing women.

Mullein

Other Names: Aaron's rod

Scientific Name: *Verbascum thapsus*

About Mullein:

Mullein is a biennial herbaceous plant with a long, upright, unbranching stem that can reach seven feet tall. It has a long taproot system. The plant is completely coated in delicate, silky hairs. The plant starts as a rosette of big, wavy-margined ovate leaves at the base.

As it matures, a flower stalk begins to develop, covered in alternate leaves that become progressively smaller up the stalk. The flower stalk is a highly distinguishing feature that grows very tall, terminating in a densely packed flower stalk, sometimes with several smaller spikes growing off the sides.

The flowers are bright yellow, each measuring just under an inch in size, with five round petals. Inside, the five stamens are usually the same yellow color but can sometimes be a dark red or purple. Each flower is replaced by a hairy green fruit capsule that turns brown when ripe.

Used For:

- Anti-inflammatory

- Antiviral

- Diuretic

- Expectorant

- Analgesic

- Tonic

- Emollient

Other Benefits:

- Decoctions are prepared from the roots of the plant to help treat sore throats and coughs.

- Poultices were made with roots and leaves by the Cherokee and Zuni tribes, to treat skin problems such as rashes, cuts, wounds, bruises, rheumatism, hemorrhoids, and athlete's foot.

- The oils from the flower are particularly beneficial for rashes and are also applied to the ears to help earache.

Medicinal Parts:

- Root

- Leaves

- Flowers

Consumed By:

- Tea made from mullein flowers and leaves is used to treat respiratory problems, colds, flu, coughs, and fevers. The leaves and roots are also smoked to help with asthma.

Possible Side Effects:

- When mullein is taken by people, there are no documented harmful side effects.

Other Important Notes:

- Mullein isn't safe for kids, pregnant women, or nursing mothers.

- The plant must be dried or processed in some way to soften the small hairs, which might otherwise cause irritation.

Thyme

Other Names: Farigoule

Scientific Name: *Thymus vulgaris*

About Thyme:

Thyme is a small branching plant that produces a variety of leaves, including the leaf base and stem base of the plant, as well as smaller green leaflets. The leaves can be small and aromatic when crushed.

Used For:

- Digestion

- Headaches

- Migraines.

Other Benefits:

- Thyme has long been known as a culinary herb. It is said to have a distinctive, pleasant fragrance that can work as an air freshener.

- It is also believed to clear the airways, making it easier for those suffering from asthma or allergies. Thyme can also be used as an antimicrobial and antiseptic.

Medicinal Parts:

- The leaves

- Flowers

- Oil

Consumed By:

- Thyme is a tea or tincture that can be taken in capsule form. It can also be made into a poultice for aches and pains.

Possible Side Effects:

- Large doses of thyme can cause stomach upset and negative side effects.

Other Important Notes:

When humans ingest it for medical purposes, there are no known harmful side effects. However, there have been some cases of skin irritation or sensitization when applied to the skin. Thyme is not recommended for children or pregnant or nursing women.

Lavender

Other Names: Mauve

Scientific Name: *Lavandula Angustifolia*

About Lavender:

Lavender is an herb that grows anywhere from 1 to 3 feet tall with small blue flowers that bloom in the summer months. It also has small pink flowers and tiny lavender-blue-colored berries. The leaves are hairy and can grow as large as 4-inch wide.

Used For:

- Stress

- Anxiety

- Depression

- Insomnia

Other Benefits:

- As this herb is also known as a culinary herb, it is widely used in cooking, flavoring, and perfumes.

- It is also said to have a distinctive, pleasant fragrance that can work as an air freshener.

- Lavender has been traditionally used to ease headaches and help promote restful sleep.

Medicinal Parts:

- Flowers

- Leaves

- Buds

Consumed By:

- Lavender is a tea or tincture that can be taken in capsule form.

- It can also be made into a poultice for aches and pains.

Possible Side Effects:

- Lavender can cause allergic reactions in people with sensitive skin.

Other Important Notes:

Lavender is not recommended for children, pregnant or nursing women due to the possible side effects.

CHAPTER THREE:
STEP 2 - ENSURE YOUR SAFETY

Now that you have gathered information about herbs, it's time to consider your safety. E is the second letter in our acronym, HEALING, and it stands for "Ensure Your Safety."This chapter will discuss the safety precautions to take when starting with herbal medicine.

So, why is ensuring your safety so important?

Herbal medicine can be very safe when properly used, but can also be very dangerous when improperly used. The majority of adverse responses to herbs are caused by improper use or failure to follow safety protocols. It's vital to remember that whatever you put in or on your body has the potential to harm you, so it's better to be cautious and safe than sorry! Luckily, herbal medicine is generally very safe and has its own guidelines and wisdom for safety.

As you consider herbs for your chronic illness or condition, you will likely have a variety of questions about safety. This chapter will address the most common concerns about using herbs to treat these conditions.

Putting together a safety plan can help you treat your illness or condition with increased confidence. A safety plan will also help you to save money in the long run. It will allow you to purchase pharmaceutical medications at reduced costs. In some cases, it's possible to choose herbal

295

alternatives that are as effective but much less expensive than pharmaceutical drugs.

If you're taking prescription and over-the-counter medications, you should be familiar with common side effects and the proper steps for managing them.

You should make sure that you understand the risks of interactions between herbal medicines and your medications. Some herbal medicines may interact with pharmaceutical drugs beneficially, but some interactions can also make your condition worse or even life-threatening.

When you find an herb that seems to be helping your conditions, read the entire label carefully to make sure you know what you're taking. Some herbs can have side effects that aren't listed on the label. If you encounter a new symptom or are concerned about something, it's best to call your doctor immediately.

Think about how these herbs might react with other medicines you take, vitamins, foods, and drinks. If you're uncertain about what might interact with a herb, it's best to ask your doctor.

If you buy herbal medicines from a health food store, consider making sure they are certified as safe as well. If you purchase them online, choose reliable sources that have security.

It's important to make sure that you have a plan for what to do if you experience side effects or reactions. While most herbal medicines are safe, some symptoms call for immediate medical attention. These symptoms include:

Swelling of the cheeks, lips, and tongue, as well as rash, hives, and dizziness. These are all examples of allergic reactions. If you have one of these symptoms after taking a herb, consult your doctor as soon as possible.

In San Francisco, two people–a man in his 50s and a woman in her 30s– were hospitalized after consuming herbal tea from a Chinatown herbalist. The plant-based poison Aconite was found in the tea leaves purchased at Sun Wing Wo Trading Company, according to the Department of Public Health. Each person developed potentially fatal irregular heart rhythms, necessitating resuscitation and extensive care (Medicalxpress, 2017).

Aconite, also known as monkshood, helmet flower, and wolfsbane is a common ingredient in Asian herbal remedies. It must be highly processed to remove toxins that can be life-threatening. Medicinal use of aconite has been traced as far back as ancient Chinese and Greek civilizations. If ingested, symptoms typically occur within 30 minutes and can include confusion, sweating, nausea, and vomiting. Severe cases may display dilated pupils, low blood pressure, slow heartbeat, and seizures.

"Symptoms can be life-threatening, and it's critically important for people to know that just a few leaves can cause them," said Dr. Tomás Aragón, San Francisco Health Officer. "Aconite poisoning can be fatal since it targets the heart" (Medicalxpress, 2017).

When purchasing herbal medicines from a store, take the time to ask about the store's policies and practices for quality control and safety. Be sure it's from a trustworthy retailer with a strong track record for customer support if you're buying something online.

Such cases of poisoning tend to make headlines, which means that many people mistakenly believe that herbal medicines are more dangerous than they actually are and opt instead to use pharmaceuticals. In reality, properly used herbs have few side effects and are much safer than pharmaceuticals. In short, herbs are safer than pharmaceuticals, but like anything else that goes into your body, there is the potential for harm.

The majority of adverse effects from herbs occur because people who are self-treating do not understand how to use the herbs properly. They believe that if a little is good, then a lot must be better.

Herbals can have a wide range of impacts on the physiological system, whereas pharmaceutical medications are more precise in their activities and illnesses they target. (Dr. Williams, 2022). There are some "drug-like" plant remedies whose effects on the human body are similar to pharmaceuticals but can be much more potent. It's critical to assess your general health and lifestyle before speaking with a healthcare professional about what you're looking for in a treatment plan. It will mean taking some time to consider your current situation before you decide on what herbal medicines you might receive.

Further research is necessary to determine whether herbal medicine is beneficial, safe, and effective for treating chronic conditions such as depression, anxiety, asthma, osteoarthritis, infectious disease, and arthritis.

Herbal medicines, overall, are aimed at healing and have a much gentler effect. Having stated that things can and do go wrong for a variety of reasons, the most common of which are:

1. Misidentification of Plants

The confusion between plants can cause a whole range of health problems. The wrong plant has a variety of effects on the human body, whereas the right one brings healing and wellbeing.

2. Incorrect Preparation

The incorrect method of preparing herbal medicines may be dangerous. The reasons include using the wrong parts of plants, using them at the wrong time of the year, or not using them with the right herbs.

3. Incorrect Administration

The wrong method of taking herbal medicines can result in the herb being taken in a way that is not effective. This can be as simple as the wrong dosage or the wrong method of ingestion, such as swallowing herbal tea leaves and herbs whole.

Herbal Medicine Side Effects

Many things can be intimidating when you're new to herbs. Understanding herbal safety is one of the most difficult areas for many new herbalists to grasp.

The truth is that herbs are extremely safe when used properly, but there are herbs with side effects. With any treatment or remedy, it is important to be aware of the potential side effects and how to deal with them.

Failure to fully research the herb you intend to use could also lead to a dangerous situation. Often, people don't know where the herbs they use come from or what method was used to harvest and process them.

Herbalism has grown in popularity, causing a huge demand for certain herbs. And since herbs are often sold as powders, tinctures, or teas, the consumer may not know exactly what they're getting until they use it.

When using herbs, it is critical to obtain the counsel of a skilled practitioner to guarantee safe use. It's also critical to calculate how much of each plant you should consume. It is not uncommon for adverse effects to occur when utilizing herbs, especially when using them for the first time. Before beginning an herb regimen, it is recommended that consumers consult with a professional.

The toxicity of the herbs can arise from the wrong dosage being given or the way it is administered. If a person is new to herbs, it is recommended that they seek out an experienced herbalist who will be able to help them with their individual situation and advise them on how to use that particular herb safely.

How to Use Herbs Safely

When choosing wild plants, you must exercise extreme caution because it is all too simple to make a mistake and pick something poisonous instead. It's easy to confuse deadly nightshade with jimson weed and dangerous toadstools with edible mushrooms, for example. If you're unsure, the best option is to get your herbs from a health food store.

1. Use the Best of the Best

So you've chosen to incorporate herbs into your family's diet, but you're not sure where to start? If you're seeking an all-natural solution, you should consult a recognized herbalist. An expert will have the expertise and tools necessary to assist you in finding the right product for your needs.

It might be tough to get high-quality herbs, especially if you're new to the herbal sector. Several new herbalists now have access to high-quality herbs, thanks to the internet. However, determining which sites are trustworthy and which are not can be challenging.

If you're not sure about a website or seller, conduct some research on their products and services before you buy anything. It is critical to learn about the seller's qualifications and certificates to assess their authenticity.

When sourcing high-quality herbs, there are 4 main factors to consider to determine what herbs are safe for your family:

1. Freshness: You must purchase your herbs from a place that uses quality packaging and has quality markers. Make sure the herbs are not expired.Herbs can stay fresh for 3-5 years. However, once they are open, there is a chance that bacteria can grow on them and make them unfit for consumption. Inspect the herbs (and packaging) for signs of spoilage.

2. Labels: When looking for herbs, you'll frequently come across terms like "natural," "organic," and "wild-crafted."

Natural Herbs - It should be noted that these are not the same thing. "Natural" is a legal term that refers to a herbal product that has not been intentionally modified to gain different effects. Many people use the term "natural" as a marketing tool, but it is important to read the label carefully before purchasing any herbal products.

Organic Herbs - Organic herbs are grown without the use of synthetic pesticides, fertilizers, or genetically modified organisms under rigorous environmental and safety conditions (GMOs). Organic herbs are grown using traditional methods, such as using low levels of pesticides and fertilizers.

Wild-crafted Herbs - These are herbs that were found in their natural state and grown as they were found. Often you will find wild-crafted herbs growing in beautiful arrays, but they can also be grown like any other herb.

3. Harvesting Practices: Another technique to assess a herb's quality is by looking into how it was harvested. Why do harvesting practices matter? Well, if the herb was harvested incorrectly, all the quality in the world won't make a difference because an improperly harvested herb is essentially useless.

Herbs should be gathered at the right time of year and with the proper equipment. Harvesting practices may be different from one herb to another, but quality herbs are always harvested using safe practices. Qualified and experienced herbalists will take their harvesting practices seriously as it directly relates to the overall quality of the product they're selling.

4. Storage: Finally, you will want to consider how herbs have been stored when purchasing. It's common for companies to freeze the herbs they harvest to maximize the preservation of their essential oils.

The quality of an herb will not matter if you're storing it improperly. If you are unable to determine how well an herb has been stored, it is probably best that you choose a different source for your herbs than what you originally intended. There are a variety of ways herbs can be stored, including freezing, refrigeration, and drying. It's crucial to figure out the best way to keep the herbs you buy because if you store them incorrectly, they may not last for a long time (Meagan, 2015).

2. Herbs are Plants...Whole Plants.

Another way to ensure safety is to use the whole plant in your preparations so that all the herb's vital components are present in your finished product. This will provide an immediate benefit but also balance and maintain your body's systems over time.

Most herbs are multipurpose, but if you want to get the maximum benefits from them, they must be used as a whole herb.

Herbs that have been fragmented or separated may contain parts that cause imbalance and disease to the body because they have been isolated from the whole plant.

Watch out for herbs that have had the chemical parts removed and only contain the isolated compound. This can be dangerous, as the isolated compound will not have co-factors that provide balance to the isolated chemical components.

Herbs can be used in different forms, but it is important to use them as a whole herb and in the correct form for your safety.

By using herbs properly, you will avoid any potential side effects and have a safe and healthy experience.

3. Herb/Drug Interactions

Herbs have been used to help the body heal on its own for many years. However, there are times when combining herbs and pharmaceuticals might aid in the treatment of sickness, but this must be done safely and healthily.

Herbs may have some extremely potent characteristics that might benefit the body, but they also have the potential to cause serious negative effects.

Some plants, for example, may mix with medicines to generate hazardous or fatal effects, according to a study. This can be a major issue for persons who are on medicine, especially when herbs are used with prescription medications.

Many herbs have a stimulant effect on the body and, if combined with others, can cause overstimulation of the system. While this may seem unpleasant for some people, it can be deadly for those taking multiple prescription drugs.

Another problem is that some herbal substances are capable of thinning the blood or reducing blood pressure and are therefore contraindicated with other herbs that also thin the blood.

To ensure safety, you need to know what types of herbs will interact with the medications you are taking. As a general rule, herbs that are said to thin the blood or reduce blood pressure should not be taken with other herbs that have the same effect.

To begin, check to see if your herb of choice interacts poorly with prescription medications. If you want to be safe, you should visit your doctor, and there are many excellent books on herbal interactions available.

Herbal interactions are not always a bad thing. If you're taking herbs and medications, it is important to consult your professional herbalist and doctor to determine if they can be safely taken together. Your herbalist or doctor will help you determine if there is an interaction between the herbs you are taking and the drugs you are taking or if there is potential for a beneficial interaction.

If you're taking prescription drugs that have the opposite effect on your herbs, a simple change in your routine may help to balance out the medicine. For example, if taking an antidepressant may be too stimulating for you, try taking it in the early morning, rather than at night time or in the evening.

4. Pharmacodynamic and pharmacokinetic interactions

Pharmacodynamic interactions can occur when herbs can interact with medications in ways that alter their effects. Pharmacodynamic interactions are those in which the herb affects how a medicine is absorbed, metabolized, or eliminated. Phytotherapy with herbs that affect the body's metabolism and the ability to eliminate drugs increases the risk of adverse effects.

Pharmacokinetic interactions can occur when herbs bind to or otherwise interfere with medicines. Pharmacokinetic interactions are those in which the herb alters the way a drug is absorbed, metabolized, or eliminated. If a medicine is bound to a herbal ingredient and the herb is ingested at the same time, it may be necessary to cut or break down the herb before taking medicine.

Herbs that contain alkaloids or other highly toxic compounds can cause serious withdrawal reactions if taken while using prescription medicines. Many of these herbs, such as ephedra, can cause severe anxiety, hallucinations, and muscle spasms if taken with certain drugs.

Aside from drug interactions, certain herbs can interact with some other herbs. For example, some herbs should not be taken with St. John's Wort at all due to their powerful mood-affecting properties.

Garlic: Garlic (Allium sativum) is a powerful antioxidant that can have many beneficial health effects on the body. But it can also interact with certain medications, including antibiotics, and it has been associated with cases of toxicity, even at relatively low doses.

Ginseng: A recent study found that ginseng (Panax species) may increase the amount of estrogen in people without a genetic predisposition or history of estrogen-related conditions. This might lead to higher blood levels of estrogen and the risk of adverse side effects.

Ginseng may also interact with medications used for high blood pressure and diabetes(NCCIH, 2022).

Kava (Piper methysticum) can interact with certain drugs, such as those used for anxiety and high blood pressure.

Combining some herbs may also increase the risk of an overdose. For example, combining dandelion with other herbs that have a diuretic effect can cause fluid loss in the body, causing dehydration and other potentially dangerous side effects, so always consult your professional herbalist and doctor if you are unsure of any potential interactions.

Herbs should not be consumed if you are taking any type of medication unless you've consulted with your doctor for their recommendations for your particular health situation.

5. Herbal Side Effects & Toxicity

While most herbs are safe to use, there are some potential side effects and toxicity that may occur with certain herbs.

- **Side Effects:** Herbs can cause side effects when they are used improperly or combined with other herbs that have an adverse effect on the body. The most common side effects of herbs include digestive problems, headaches, and bloating.

For example, if you decide to take black cohosh together with a diuretic like valerian root, this can interfere and cause unexpected results. Making sure you know what herbs your body will tolerate is important to avoid any potential problems.

Herbs that cause the most side effects include Birthwort, Comfrey, and Senna. These herbs are known to cause severe digestive problems, electrolyte abnormalities, and excessive uterine bleeding.

Herbs like Angelica and Chaparral, on the other hand, might be harmful to your health since they contain poisonous compounds that can harm your liver. It is critical to seek medical advice before utilizing these herbs.

- **Toxicity:** Sometimes, when you take herbs, it is necessary to do so in larger amounts than what you might normally use. This is especially true with some of the more potent herbs.

If something goes wrong and the herb does cause a toxic reaction, it is essential to contact your herbalist and institute an emergency plan for treatment to keep your health as stable as possible.

Because the body doesn't create as many enzymes for breaking down these herbs, as well as a decrease in saliva production, if a person takes too much of a herb, the excess amount of herbs held in the body might make them hazardous.

Being aware that herbs can be toxic and how they are used can help you understand how the effects of herbs can affect your health. It's critical to understand which herbs are beneficial or harmful to you and your health.

How To Test Herbs For Allergic Reactions

Are you aware that some herbs can cause an allergic reaction? Yes, some herbs can cause an allergic reaction, and these reactions can be very serious for some people.

If you're experiencing an allergic reaction to an herb, it is important to stop using the herb immediately and contact your professional herbalist and doctor if necessary.

There are some side effects of herbs related to allergies. If you're allergic to any type of herb, your professional herbalist should be able to advise you on possible alternatives or the appropriate herbs that can be taken.

Certain herbs are more common allergens than other herbs, and many people are allergic to the same plant in different ways.

While several allergies are direct reactions to an allergen in the herb, some allergies may not be evident at first sight.

Testing for allergic reactions is important for your health, but it can also be difficult and frustrating if you're not sure what herbs you may be allergic to.

1. Start by pressing the fresh herb on the inside of your wrist's skin and waiting for a skin reaction before drinking it. If you only have dry herbs, soak them in warm water for a few minutes and then rub the wet herb on your skin. Continue to 'Step 2' if no reaction occurs.

2. Take 1 teaspoon of a strong herbal infusion. 30 minutes later, try again if you notice no reaction.

3. Drink 1/2 cup after 30 min if no reaction is noticed.

4. Wait a few minutes more, and then test a full cup.

If no reaction is still observed, then you are most likely not allergic to the herb.

It's important to remember that you can be allergic to an herb even if you weren't previously allergic to it, or vice versa. It's also possible that someone is allergic to a component of the herb that they previously tolerated.

In general, if your reaction to herbs changes suddenly, you should contact your herbalist. If you're trying an herb for the first time, start small and work your way up to bigger doses if you're comfortable.

If you do experience a reaction, it should go away after about 1 day. If not, it is important to contact your herbalist or doctor to find out what is going on and what you can do about it.

Test all herbs again after 2 weeks to see if any allergic reaction occurs again before starting taking the herb regularly.

Determining Herbal Dosages

Herbal dosage guides are given in the form of a 'potency' or 'potency range'. Potency is a wide range of doses that defines the effects of an herb. Dosage levels may vary based on various factors:

1. Weight - Most herbs have been tested and standardized based on a 150-pound adult. So when giving a child an herbal remedy, you may need to reduce the dosage accordingly.

2. Nutritional vs. Medicinal Use - Herbs that are given for nutritional purposes aren't necessarily given in the same amount as when they're intended for medicinal use.

3. Acute vs. Chronic Ailments - Herbal preparations given to treat acute conditions, such as a cold or the flu are generally given in larger amounts than those given for chronic conditions. The reason for this is that herbs may need to be taken for longer periods for chronic ailments, and so their dosage needs to be sufficient.

4. Method of Preparation - The method of preparation– if it is a decoction or infusion–also affects the dosage, as small adjustments may be necessary. An example of this is with root herbs.The decoction method allows for tougher plant material (roots and bark) or a larger amount to be steeped and herbal potency to be increased.

Decoctions are particularly effective for herbs that need to be boiled for a long time to extract their medicinal properties. You can make decoctions with several different herbs, and they can range from needing a few minutes to 12 hours of steeping. After the herb has simmered, then the liquid is strained through a cloth.

You may also want to experiment and look up information on the internet on your chosen herb to find out more information on dosage.

5. Fresh vs. Dried - The potency of an herb can vary based on how it was grown and harvested. Fresh herbs tend to be stronger than dried herbs.

6. Farmed vs. Wild - Herbs that aren't wild-crafted are cultivated. And while most herbalists tend to stick with cultivated herbs, the dosage of these herbs may be different than those that are wild-crafted.

7. Menstruum Used - Dried herbs (such as flowers, leaves, and roots) are typically placed in a 'menstruum' that helps with the extraction of the herb's medicinal properties. However, when using fresh plants, you may need to make a menstruum yourself from a brine that has 1 part fresh water to 1 part sea salt.

If the dosage of your herbal remedy is not adequate for your use, you may want to increase it at home by using an appropriate herbal essence.

Herbal essences are used to increase the medicinal properties of an herb, and they are typically added to the menstruum before steeping.

One of the most common herbal essences used is a tincture, which is made by soaking an herb in a menstruum, such as alcohol.

8. Maceration Time - The duration of time that herbs are macerated in a menstruum can affect the medicinal properties and healing abilities. If an herb is macerated for too long, the strength of its medicinal properties will be diluted. But if a macerate and herb are steeped too long, it can get bitter (Meagan, 2015).

Methods Of Determining Herbal Dosage

A great way to determine the proper dosage is to follow the recommendations of a practitioner. A herbalist or naturopath can give you an idea of how much to take. Some practitioners may also be able to recommend a specific dosage for you on your initial visit. You can also ask them about dosages for general health purposes, whether morning or night, active or resting periods, or any other factors that may have an effect on your health and well-being.

When you come across a herbal cure, you'll usually find the method of preparation first, followed by the dose amount. This is perfect because the dosage has already been delivered to you. However, you may encounter difficulties due to a lack of knowledge on how much to take. In this situation, you can choose from one of the following four options:

1. Include a Disclaimer - This method is simple and effective. Simply include a disclaimer that states, "This herbal medicine should not be taken more than this dose amount or for longer than this period." Simply include your practitioner's or alternative health specialist's advice in your list.

2. Minimalist Approach (Titrate Dosing) - This method is when you start out with a small dosage, and then you increase the dosage amount while monitoring your health until you reach the desired effect.

3. Folk Method Dosing - Another popular dosing method used among alternative health practitioners is the folk method of dosing. Giving 1 drop for every 2 pounds of body weight as a starting point and then titrating the dose as mentioned above is how this approach, which uses 50 % alcohol or glycerin, works.

4. Children's Formulas - Many people find it hard to figure out the proper dosage of an herbal remedy for children. One such way to determine the dosage is to use a child-friendly formula.

The following two rules may also be helpful when figuring out the proper dosage:

- **Fried's Rule:** - Calculate the adult dose by multiplying the child's age in months by 150.

- **Clark's Rule:** - Calculate the adult dose by multiplying the child's weight in pounds by 150.

Who Shouldn't Use Herbal Medicine?

Herbal medicine is not for every person or for every condition. You should not use herbal medicine if you have the following:

- Medical conditions, including cancer - You should talk to your medical professional when considering supportive herbal remedies when you have a serious condition such as cancer.

- Undergoing Chemotherapy- If you are having chemotherapy an herbal regime can be and is more frequently used to provide support to your immune system and manage the side effects of treatment. Make sure you are transparent with your medical professionals and with your natural medicine practitioners, so they can guide you on your course of action.

- Pregnant or Breastfeeding - While there is no evidence to show that herbal medicine can harm the health of an unborn or breastfeeding infant, it is better to be safe than sorry. If you're pregnant or nursing, talk to your doctor before starting a herbal medication program.

If you are having surgery in the next few weeks - You should wait at least two to three weeks before starting any herbal formula. If you have any surgery planned, you should consult with your physician before taking herbal medicine.

- Children - You should not use herbal medicine on children under 14 years of age unless it is with the recommendation of a physician and/or alternative health professional.

- Elderly - It is advised that elderly people see a physician before using herbal medicine.

With that said, most herbal medicine is safe when used correctly. You just have to be mindful of the potential side effects and limitations on who can use them.

Chapter Four:
Step 3 - Acquire Your Herbs

Having ensured safety in the preparation and use of herbal medicine, it is now time to acquire the herbs you will be using to make the herbal medicine. In our HEALING framework, the letter A which stands for "Acquire Your Herbs," is our third step to getting into Herbal Medicine.

Acquiring your herbs means acquiring the herbs you will be using to make your herbal medicine, in other words, getting the proper plants for your medicine so that you can begin the Herbal Medicine recipe.

This chapter will enlighten you on the importance of properly sourcing your herbs and how to make sure you are getting high-quality herbs that are effective and safe.

The first thing you need to know about gathering herbs is that not all herbs are harvested in the same way. Some herbs are harvested commonly, while others require skill and effort to harvest.

Most complaints about herbal medicine not working may simply be due to the lack of potency of the herbs you have. Sourcing your herbs carefully is crucial in ensuring you have safe, potent, and effective remedies.

When you take herbal medicine, it is important that you only take high-quality, potent herbs. Proper sourcing will ensure that your herbal remedies are backed by science and expert knowledge when it comes to their effectiveness, safety, and potency.

Herbs should be of high quality as a rule. The higher the quality of the herb, the better the medicinal value.

In the Netflix documentary, *Broken*, they tell a story about fake cosmetics that contained toxic ingredients. The film discusses how important it is to know where your items come from and whether they are from a reputable source. Realizing that your face cream is from a trusted source through a little research will go a long way (Morgan, 2016). Counterfeit cosmetics are knockoffs of well-known brands sold at swap meetings, street markets, and some online marketplaces.

You may be getting a deal, but you might not be getting the authentic products or the high-quality products you think - they could have been fake. The companies that make these counterfeit products look like they're experts at creating knockoffs, but they cut costs and corners by using toxic ingredients that are potentially harmful to your health.

Going to the source of your product can mean the difference between an effective, safe, and quality product and not. You don't want to be known as the person who bought a fake face cream. You want to know who, what, where, when, and why you're investing your hard-earned cash.

Whether buying bulk dried herbs, herbs in packets, or tinctures, make sure your herbs are of the highest quality. You should always look for organic herbs and be sure to get them from a reputable source.

The lack of regulation of herbal medicine can cause serious health problems. There have been instances of people using contaminated herbs, leading to serious health problems that could have been avoided. Essentially, you do not want to be the victim of a "bad batch" or a counterfeit product. The inconsistent quality across all sellers of herbal medicine can make it hard to identify whether you are getting a high-quality, safe product or not.

Look for brands that have been tested for quality by a third-party organization (US Pharmacopeia or NSF International) and, ideally, have science-based customer reviews that can be used as a reference for the quality of the product.

When buying bulk herbs in bulk containers, ensure that the container is properly sealed. This can ensure you are not getting stale herbs from an earlier date. Also, make sure to see the expiration date and also purchase from reputable brands or companies where you can reach a qualified customer service representative to answer your questions and help you if anything should arise.

Signs of High-Quality Herbal Medicines

When sourcing your herbs, look for the following signs of high-quality herbs that can be used to make your herbal remedies:

1. Choose The Correct Herb

Research the herbs you are taking or consult with a herbal practitioner. To make the best use of the herb, you have to have the right herb in the right amount. Not all remedies are made for all people or ailments. If one is taking herbs for constipation, then you may want to avoid some herbs that may cause intestinal upset, particularly those with large amounts of magnesium. Know which parts of the plant have the desired medicine and how it is taken before you buy the herb.

These herbal parts have different therapeutic uses and should be taken differently. For example, stinging nettle roots and leaves contain an anti-inflammatory chemical and steroid response, but the roots contain more steroid-like substances.

2. Harvested at Their Peak

To get the most potent medicine, different plant parts should be gathered at different stages of the plant's growth. This is when the majority of the medicine is formed.

The Leaves and Stems: Harvest just before the plant flowers for the highest concentration of medicine.

The Flowering Heads: Harvest flowering Eurasian water-milfoil when in full bloom for the highest concentration of medicine. It's a general rule that flowers should be harvested just before or during the height of their bloom.

The Roots and Rhizomes: Harvest when a new crown grows, like at the end of each growing season. This is how to get a potent harvest from roots like garlic or ginger.

3. Use the Most Potent Plant Parts

The fact that a plant is medicinal does not imply that the entire plant is medicinal or that all parts of the plant have the same therapeutic use.

For example, the leaf, stem, and flower of dandelion are medicinal, but each part is used for very different purposes. The root of the dandelion contains a lot more medicine than the stem and leaves.

4. Herbs are Sold by a Reputable Company

Another sign of high-quality herbs is that they are sold by a reputable company. Reputable companies will be more likely to use high-quality herbs because they want repeat business and won't want you to go elsewhere. Reputable companies may also have science-based customer reviews and other ways to assure you of their knowledge and quality products.

Examples of reputable companies include:

- Bulkherbstore https://www.bulkherbstore.com/

- Mountainroseherbs https://mountainroseherbs.com/

- Frontier Co-op   http://www.frontiercoop.com/

- Pacific Botanicals http://www.pacificbotanicals.com/

- Oregon's Wild Harvest
  https://www.oregonswildharvest.com/

- The Herb Academy
  https://theherbalacademy.com/purchase-herbs-
  and-supplies-world-wide/

5. Right Preparation Methods

Be on the lookout for inconsistent methods of preparation. Some herbs can be taken raw, but most need to be dried or powdered to use them. Always look for an active ingredient rather than just an herb. The reason most people choose a herbal remedy is that they believe it will work better than conventional medicines and drugs, so they want a safe, potent product that works.

When buying your herbs, look at the number of active ingredients or medicinal properties in each product. The more you can find in the product, the better it is for you.

The processing of herbs is just as important as the picking. Different methods of processing, grinding, and drying can affect the quality and concentration of the medicinal properties in your product. While some plants need to be dried for better efficacy, other plants are sensitive to heat and should never be cooked.

6. Plants are Contaminant Free

Another good sign that you are buying high-quality herbs is to ensure they are free of pesticides, insecticides, and herbicides. These chemicals can alter the natural properties of the plants and may cause harm to your body.

7. Freshness

Ensure that the herbs you buy are fresh. If your product has been sitting out for too long, it will be more likely to lose its potency.

8. Storage

Lastly, always make sure you store your herbs in a dry, cool place. This can prevent the herbs from losing their potency (Carolyn, 2019).

Foraging For Herbs

Buying is not your only option for sourcing herbs. Foraging is a type of gathering or hunting that involves the practice of collecting wild plants and exploring the landscape by finding edible plants. It is a very useful skill to have because you can find all sorts of amazing herbs in your neighborhood.

When foraging for herbs, you should always be careful about what you bring home and make sure it is legal to harvest. So before you start foraging, do your research.

Foraging for herbs can be a great way to ensure you are getting good-quality herbal medicine. Foraging for herbs can give you access to the most potent ones that are growing near you and make them more easily accessible.

Herbs commonly found in our backyards and local parks or forests could be used by an herbalist, but recently many people have been using them as cheaper alternatives to pharmaceuticals and over-the-counter medications.

Herb foraging can be a terrific way to get the most effective and safe plants possible, but it can be challenging. Herbs can often be found growing near you, but several are more common in more populous places. Despite this, there are still certain ways to forage for some of these powerful herbs.

Foraging for wild herbs is far less reliable as a source of supply than many people believe.

Herbal species are often only found by accident in undisturbed areas, and because they are not grown in a protected garden, they are far more likely to be contaminated with pesticides or badly managed.

Foraging also relies on being physically close to the plant you want to harvest, as well as being able to identify it correctly. This is one reason why wild-crafting is best done in your own habitat.

Foraging is also a more time-consuming tactic, and it is, therefore, best used as a last resort.

There are different ways of sourcing plants from where they grow naturally, but only the best techniques must be used. This is important for ensuring that natural bushes and forests are not depleted.

By best technique is meant the methods that ensure both the herb users and the environment can continue to benefit from human activity. If the methods used are inappropriate, where people harvest herbs without concern as to what happens to the environment, soon future generations could be unable to find natural herbs to use for either food or natural healing.

Harvesting Shrubby Plants

If the plant you want for your medicine is a shrub and the part you want is either a branch or the stem, ensure the spot you aim to cut is above a leaf node. This is crucial because from that leaf node will emerge another branch or stem, and the plant continues to thrive.

There should be 6 millimeters between the leaf node and where you make your cut. Your cut should be diagonal, at an angle of 45°. The only time you may cut right across is if the plant you are getting your piece of herb from has two leaves exactly opposite each other on that spot.

Replanting

Whenever you harvest an herb, pick its root crown and replant it whenever that is possible. This will hopefully produce more plants of that species where you found it. Not all plants are suitable for replanting, therefore you must do your research before replanting.

Timing

If you intend to source your herbal medicine from a root, make a point of harvesting your roots during the fall season. The reason for this is that leaves fall off their mother plants in the fall, or they just die. When this happens, the majority of nutrients wind up in the roots of the plant.

Not only are you bound to harvest potent roots, but any remaining roots are likely to continue becoming strong faster and grow again the next season.

Starting with Broken Branches

Harvest any branches that have broken off and are hanging from the plant first. By so doing, you will have accomplished your mission of getting herbs for use, and beyond that, you will have protected the plant from possible infection.

So, to reduce the chances of the plant developing a disease cut off that broken branch in a manner that flattens the broken surface.

How to Cut a Branch Safely

If you want to cut off a tree branch, begin by cutting it to a depth of two inches on its underside. Then continue cutting from the top side.The reason is that while the bark of the tree is safe at the top surface because you continue sawing deep into the tree, you run the risk of peeling off the bark on the underside if you do not have a ready-cut beneath.

In short, you want to cut off the branch you need for your use but leave the tree with its bark intact; and not partly stripped.

How to Gather Medicinal Herbs

It is important to understand the dos and don'ts of wild-crafting, where wild-crafting stands for harvesting herbal plants from their natural habitat for medicinal use.

People from ancient cultures carried out wild-crafting in their time and used the plants as sources of medicine and also as important ingredients during particular rituals.

Although these uses have continued for many centuries, there are still medicinal herbs available for use in forests and bushes; the reason being that the people concerned have continued their herb harvesting responsibly.

It is, therefore, important to learn how best to go about harvesting herbs for medicinal use so these herbs do not become extinct. It would undoubtedly be great if future generations could benefit from herb-based natural treatments the way others before them have done.

Spare endangered plants

First of all, make a point of sparing any species of herb you know to be endangered. This will help it to flourish and be available for use sometime in the future.

Identify plants correctly

Identify the right plant species by comparing descriptions and notes that appear in various books and sources, such as photographs.

Do not harvest plants randomly. One reason for this is that you run the risk of consuming a poisonous herb if you mistakenly pick the wrong plant. Some herbs resemble one another, and it only takes one or two features, sometimes subtle or inconspicuous, to differentiate them.

Another reason is that if you pick the herb you did not intend to, you probably will end up discarding it, and that will be an unnecessary waste.

Avoid highly placed plants

There is good reason to avoid the plants on very high ground, which are usually far more mature than the rest—repopulation.

Often you will be harvesting your herbs from land that is slanting and rising in gradient as you move up. Once you avoid moving to the peak, you let those mature plants drop seeds to areas below where more herbs can continue growing. In short, the herb harvesting area should be somewhere below the top areas where mature plants are mostly established.

Also, choose the plants with several healthy branches. This is because you must leave the plant strong and healthy and in a position to produce more branches and continue thriving.

You should do the same if you are targeting leaves as well. You must leave the plant with sufficient leaves to make food for the plant and to play the other roles plant leaves do within the habitat.

One important principle you need to adhere to is ensuring that what you pick from a single plant does not exceed 10% of what that plant has. This is responsible and respectful wild-crafting.

Bring the Accurate Tools

If you want to harvest, be sure you have the appropriate equipment for the task. The following tools will enable you to achieve this goal:

Bags or Baskets: Bags or baskets help you collect the leaves and flowers of plants. You can use a simple bag made of cloth to collect plant leaves and also to keep them together. These bags can be used for both urban and rural wild-crafting, and they are often quite affordable. You'll be able to collect a significant quantity of leaves at once without needing to move from one location to another.

Pruning Shears and Scissors: Pruning shears come in handy when you want to harvest branches. Scissors can be useful if you want to pick leaves, but it is always important you use the right scissor for the right plant.

*A **Field Guide:*** A field guide can help you identify plants with full accuracy and avoid confusion at a later date. These guides are great tools for identifying and distinguishing between herbs when they come into use, especially if more than one species of a given herb exists in the habitat.

*A **Strong Stick for Digging:*** A stick will help you dig out the root of a herb. If you have ever dug up a plant, you will realize that it is necessary to dig down until you find the center and then pull it out.

*A **Paper and Pen:*** It is always helpful to have paper and a pen with you, even when going herb picking. This will enable you to note down the details of the herbs you picked and also the location where you picked them from. You can use this information to help others in your community or family with similar needs in the future (Meagan, 2015).

Always make sure you have appropriate clothes on while harvesting. This will help ensure that you are comfortable, protected from the elements, and safe from potential threats.

As always, make sure to keep in mind common sense when wild-crafting. Always make sure you can do the task before proceeding. Wild-crafting might be a fun activity for some, but harvesting herbs for medicinal purposes is serious business.

Growing Herbs Yourself

Growing your own herbs may be a rewarding and enjoyable experience. It will not only save you money, but it will also ensure that you get high-quality herbs because you will be in charge of how they are cultivated.

Buying herbs you need can be costly during some seasons, especially if you rely on going to the market for most of your herbal needs.

It is worth considering growing them yourself to avoid the high costs associated with buying herbs from the market every time you need them.

Growing herbs can be done in many ways, depending on the type of herb you want to grow.

If you want to grow herbs for medicinal purposes (not simply for decoration), then it is important to choose an herbal garden with an appropriate climate in which they will thrive.

The most common garden that is widely used is the medicinal one. These gardens are usually located near where the herbs will be harvested, and they typically use a variety of methods to ensure the plants thrive and produce high-quality herbs.

Here are some detailed basics of growing herbs at home, at your convenience, and on a schedule you choose.

Finding Herbs To Grow

Acquiring herbs can be done in two principal ways:

1. Find pre-grown plants - You have different options at your disposal when it comes to finding pre-grown herbs. For example, you can go to the local farmer's market and choose to buy plants that are already grown. Also, you can visit other people who have grown herbs and ask them if they would be willing to give or sell some of their plants (in case they have more than they can use). Another option is to go out in search of any wild plants that grow around your area and choose those.

Before you plant a herb, it is important to check the conditions needed for its growth. The weather conditions, the soil type, and how it's watered are all things you should consider before planting any herb.

2. Growing Herbs Seeds Yourself - Growing herbs from seeds is a less expensive way of getting started. It can also help you better understand the specific growing conditions needed for each type of herb. All you need to do is purchase organic herb seeds from your local grocery store or on the internet. Plants can be started from seed in a variety of ways, but before you get started, do some research on the herb you want to cultivate, so you know its needs. Some plants, for example, do not like to be transplanted from seed pots, so they must be sown directly where they will grow.

When you're ready to plant the herb seeds, use a container that is at least 4 inches in depth. If the soil is too dry, there won't be enough moisture for the seeds to take root, so make sure to thoroughly water before planting. If you notice that the soil is too wet, remove some of the top layers before planting. It is important to remember that after you see roots coming through the bottom of your soil container, it is time to transplant them into a larger container. As the plant grows and outgrows its current pot, it is important to maintain good drainage for the plant, so it doesn't get root-bound.

Note: Starting from pre-grown plants is easier than growing from a seed, but unless you are planning to harvest only a few herbs, buying herb plants is usually more expensive than starting from seed.

It's also prudent to keep in mind that the more you buy at once, the cheaper it will be.

After harvesting your herbs, storing them is essential. You want to make sure they are properly stored to ensure that they stay fresh and ready for use at a future date.

Hanging them up in bunches with a string or rubber band is a good way to store fresh herbs for several days. Most herbs can be stored for up to one week this way.

If you need your herbs for medicinal purposes, proper storage will help you preserve them longer so you can enjoy their benefits.

You can store harvested herbs in several ways. You can keep them in a container with a tight lid (preferably glass), or you can freeze them in a plastic bag with an unsealed end that you can use to remove the herbs you need later on. Keep in mind that this method may result in some loss of flavor and aroma because of the effect of cold temperatures on the volatile essential oils found in plants.

The powdered form of herbs can be stored in a container with a tight lid. Just remember that the longer dry herbs are stored, the greater their chance of becoming stale and losing their flavor.

Your prepared remedies can also be stored in a glass jar or other container with a tight lid. Then you can use them as needed.

Chapter Five:
Step 4 - Learn the Methods of Preparation

After acquiring your high-quality herbal medicine, you will need to learn the methods that are used to make the remedies.

This brings us to the letter **L**, the fourth in our acronym of how to get into herbal medicine, which stands for the *"Learn Method of Preparation."*

In this chapter, we will learn about the methods that are used to make herbal medicines and the equipment necessary for preparing them.

This chapter will help you get into making your own herbal remedies. You can use your herbs, or you can use commercially prepared ones as well. Either way, it's important to know how to do so to increase your proficiency in using herbal remedies safely and effectively.

In the modern world we live in, people are often preoccupied with getting more done as quickly and efficiently as possible. This can lead to a tendency to take shortcuts when it comes to preparing medicines.

There is nothing wrong with wanting to make the most of your time, but if you are not careful and do not know what you're doing, you can accidentally ingest or inhale irritating chemicals such as formaldehyde, ammonia, or alcohol.

You may find yourself drinking something that should be applied topically only or applying a salve or balm to the wrong part of your body.

Don't laugh, it has happened and will continue to happen to those who are not paying attention or are in a hurry.

But if you learn how to prepare herbal medicines the right way, you will be able to avoid these mishaps and take advantage of all that Mother Nature has given us.

Preparation–Essential Tools

With all that said, let's list some of the essential tools that will be useful in preparing herbal medicines and remedies:

- **Food Scale** - You will use the food scale to measure herbs, roots, and powders both for liquid and dry remedies such as capsules. Get one that measures in both ounces and grams, as most recipes call for both measurements.

- **Mortar and Pestle** - A mortar and pestle are essential for grinding herbs to obtain their purest forms.

This tool is also useful for crushing plant material into a fine powder.

It's also possible to crush or grind non-herbal materials using a mortar and pestle, but you should always do so with utmost caution.

337

- **Quart Sized Mason Jars** - Mason jars are handy for storing herbs and ingredients for your remedies. You can use them for both dry and liquid remedies.

- **Pint-Sized Mason Jars** - These are also very useful for storing herbs. You can use pint-sized jars to hold herbs that you will be using to make salves and other herbal products that require a thicker consistency.

Pint-sized jars can also be used to store remedies that have been strained after infusion.

- **3 Quart Crock Pot** - You will need a crockpot to make herbal teas, infusions, and decoctions.

You should also get a timer to help you know when it is time to turn the heat off and let your remedy cool down.

Most recipes call for the use of a crockpot.

Note: The more volatile the herb you choose, the more important it is that you use either a crockpot or double broiler method instead of boiling on the stovetop.

- **6 Quart Crockpot** - If you plan on making large batches of herbal remedies, or if you have a larger family, a 6-quart crockpot is the way to go.

Most recipes require a 4-quart crock pot, so find the best fit for yourself.

- **Magic Bullet** - A Magic Bullet is a handy tool for blending herbs and making herbal extracts.

It also comes in handy for chopping, grinding, and pureeing herbs.

You can use the same Magic Bullet for making herbal extracts as well as some of your herbal remedies, but you should not use the same one to do both at the same time.

- **Coffee Grinder** - This can be helpful if you want to grind your herbs into a powder to make capsules with.

You can also use the coffee grinder to grind other non-herbal ingredients to save time on food preparation.

You may also need a hand grinder for grinding herbs that are too hard or tough for a standard coffee grinder.

- **Stainless Steel Saucepans** - These are used to prepare herbal extracts and remedies that require simmering. For liquid remedies, you should use stainless steel instead of aluminum for the best results.

Stainless steel will also hold heat longer than aluminum and will not give off aluminum particles that are toxic to the body. Get 1, 2, and 4-quart saucepans, as well as small and medium-sized saucepans.

A variety of stainless steel pots will ensure that you are prepared for whatever you may need to prepare.

- **Double Boiler** - This is a very useful tool for preparing herbal remedies.

You can use it to boil your tea and other herbal remedies.

It is also convenient for heating other ingredients for making soups and mixtures to avoid having to use a stovetop.

- **Tea Kettle** - The tea kettle is useful for all kinds of herbal teas, including herbal decoctions, infusions, and tisanes.

A tea Kettle can be used safely on a stovetop.

You will also need an extra tea kettle for making herbal extracts to keep the herbs from burning.

Stainless steel is the best material for tea kettles because it is non-reactive and will not leach metals into your tea.

- **Funnels** - Funnels are essential for any kitchen, especially when it comes to herbs.

Funnels are useful for transferring ingredients from one container to another without spilling or making a mess.

- **Cheesecloth** - This is a cheap alternative to using coffee filters to strain your herbal remedies.

Cheesecloth is also useful for straining out unwanted seeds and fibers from your tea or herbal remedies.

- **Natural Parchment Paper** - This is a kind of parchment paper that you can use instead of regular paper.

Natural parchment paper is very durable and will not burn or melt when making herbal remedies.

It is also non-reactive, meaning it will not leach any metals into your herbal remedies.

- **Stainless steel mixing bowls** - These are used for making herbal remedies such as infusions and decoctions.

You will also need a stainless steel bowl for straining your herbal remedies.

I recommend using either 1 or 4-quart bowls, depending on how much you plan on preparing at a time.

This will allow you to use the same bowl over and over again instead of needing to purchase new ones every time you make a new remedy.

- **Glass Mixing Bowls** - Glass mixing bowls are very versatile.

You can use them to make herbal extracts, decoctions, infusions, and other herbal remedies.

Glass is non-reactive, so it will not leach metals into your herbal remedies.

- **Stainless Measuring Cups** - use a variety of stainless steel measuring cups, starting with a ¼-cup.

They are useful for making sure that you get the right amount of herbs in your herbal remedies.

- **Stainless Measuring spoons** - You should have a set of measuring spoons with ¼, ½, 1, and 1 ½-teaspoon measures. Make sure they are made out of stainless steel or glass so they will not leach any metals into your herbal remedies.

- **2 cup Glass Measuring Cup** - This is very handy for measuring out water, other ingredients, and melted substances for making remedies.

- **Wooden spoons** - These are very useful for stirring, mixing, and cooking with herbs.

You will also need a small wooden spoon for measuring out the correct amount of water and fresh herbs for making herbal infusions.

Wood is inert, so it will not leach any toxic substances into your herbal remedies.

- **Silicone spatulas** - These can be used to scrape up any lingering herbs in your pot or pan after making your herbal remedies.

- **Notebook** - This is handy for writing out your recipes and making notes.

Notebooks can also be used to take notes on supplements, herbs, and other herbal remedies.

- **Labels** - Use sticker labels to label your jars and bottles when storing your herbal remedies.

Labels are helpful because they will allow you to identify which of your remedies are which.

This is especially helpful if you have a large number of remedies or mixtures and want to keep them organized.

- **Permanent Marker** - You will need this to label your bottles, jars, and other containers.

Markers are also useful for labeling your herbal ingredients to keep them organized.

You should use black permanent markers rather than dry-erase markers because of the long-term use that is required.

- **Metal Tins** - Metal tins can be used to store your herbs, spices, and other ingredients.

They are especially useful for storing dried herbs that contain volatile oils because they will prevent the oils from evaporating.

- **Colored Tincture Bottles** - These are useful for storing your tinctures.

Note: Only glass containers should be used for storing herbal remedies, as metal and plastic may leach harmful substances into your herbal remedies.

- **Muslin Bags** - Muslin bags can be used to filter out herbs that are not suitable for your herbal remedies.

Muslin bags are also useful as a way to strain out undesirable seeds and fibers from your herbal remedies.

- **Essential Oils** - Essential oils are used for therapeutic purposes and can be added to many herbal remedies.

Look for essential oils that are certified organic, pure, and unadulterated.

You can also use essential oils as a way to store your herbal remedies.

Adding the correct amount of essential oil—as listed on the dosage label—to your preparation will prevent it from spoiling.

Most of these above-listed items are probably available in your home kitchen already, but it is always good to have a set of your own. You never know when you may need them and having your own set will make it easier to find them quickly.

A few of the above-listed items can be found in your local grocery store, but most are only available through specialty shops. Sometimes you will be able to find everything you need in your local grocery store, but keep in mind that natural remedies are not often stocked at your local grocery store. The best way to find what you need is to check out your local natural foods store and its online outlets (Meagan, 2015).

Why Is Preparation Important?

Processing your herbs properly is the most important step in the whole herbal remedy-making process. It is how you prepare your herbs that will determine how effective your herbal remedies are.

Preparation helps to preserve the potency of your herbs, so your remedies will last longer. Preparation is also the most important step because you will want your herbal remedies to be effective as soon as possible. The sooner you start using them, the sooner you can reap the benefits.

Another good reason to focus on the quality of preparation is that it helps to remove any unwanted materials and contaminants. Those contaminants can be toxic and have an adverse effect on your body. This is especially important when making herbal remedies that you will be ingesting or using on your skin.

If you are working with a recipe, then the preparation steps will be noted in the instructions. However, certain general guidelines or considerations should be followed when working with herbs in any capacity and preparing them for herbal remedies.

Many of the herbs you harvest are meant to provide medications in varying forms, such as decoctions, tinctures, and others. You, therefore, need to know how to go about preparing the medications in their different forms.

Methods of Preparation

There are various ways to prepare herbal remedies, each with pros and cons. These methods have been meticulously developed over the ages through a tedious process of trial and error and have been used by human beings for health and wellness purposes for centuries.

Herbalists have studied the therapeutic properties of plants and determined that each portion of a plant has its unique medicinal properties, with varying degrees of efficacy in various forms. Some plants, for example, are more effective when used in oils, whereas others are more effective when used in tinctures. The way you prepare your herbal treatments has a big impact on how effective they are.

Before making your herbal treatments, it's usually a good idea to do some research. While this book is a good starting point, it wouldn't hurt to do some additional study to be sure you're not mixing herbs that aren't meant to be mixed together. It takes a lot of patience, trial, and error to figure out which technique of preparation works best for which herb and what amounts and dosages make for optimal effectiveness while avoiding side effects.

Aside from online research, visiting local herbal or health food stores to observe how they package various herbs is a smart method. Similar herbs will be put together on shelves so that you can see what properties and actions they have in common. You can also check the label for recommended dosages to see how much you should take safely.

In this chapter, you will learn what constitutes the different herbal remedies and get tips on how you can make these remedies and recipes by yourself at home. Each method has a different level of potency, which will be mentioned, so you can tell which is the strongest and fastest acting and which are gentler versions of the remedies.

The measurements may differ depending on the use, but make sure you don't exceed the suggested dosage. Before you use the herbs, find out how strong they are and what effects they have. You shouldn't utilize any herbs you're not familiar with because you won't know how they interact with others or your body.

The part of the herb that you use also makes a big difference. The leaves, roots, stems, seeds, and flowers all carry different actions, so you might need to adjust the amount you are using in accordance with the part of the herb.

A good rule of thumb is to use one ounce of any singular herb or one ounce of combined herbs. If you are using dried herbs, you would need to use twice the amount as you would fresh herbs.

These herbal remedies can be made with either dried or fresh herbs. Consider growing your own herbs to save money if you have the space. You can even wild-craft herbs if you develop a keen eye for them.

One thing to remember when deciding which herbal method you should use is that you need to decipher which part of the body they are needed for. How can you get the herbs you want as close to the area of the body where you need them, and as efficiently as you possibly can.

For example, if you have a splinter in your foot, you wouldn't consider drinking herbal tea to see if it can pop out as a result; you'd work on getting the splinter out directly by yourself. You'd analyze the area; "the splinter is on my foot, and I can pull it out using a pair of tweezers." A similar principle applies to working with herbal remedies as well. For instance, if you have a headache you can make a soothing and pain-relieving poultice that you can apply directly on the forehead for pain relief.

How effective our herbs are depends on how well their gradual action restores the natural balance of your body's natural, healthy functions. It is very seldom that herbal remedies are capable of producing long-lasting beneficial effects after just one dose. You need to continue taking the remedy to have long-lasting results.

If you are treating a chronic problem with herbal remedies, generally, it would take a month of herbal treatments to treat each year that you have suffered from the problem. For example, if you have suffered from chronic backache for five years, it would take at least five months of herbal remedies to treat that problem.

When you're making herbal preparations using medicinal herbs, you need to make sure that any treatments that you consume are prepared fresh every day. This rule doesn't apply to herbal salves, ointments, liniments, and tinctures, as you can keep them stored properly for long periods. It would be best to keep things as simple as possible to avoid overcomplicating things and risking an adverse reaction. Try using one herb at a time in the beginning until you get the hang of things and you can combine different herbs effectively.

As there are so many types of preparation methods, measurement is incredibly important. Overusing any medicinal herb can be detrimental to your health, so it is essential that you learn how to properly mix your solutions; this is a cardinal rule of alternative medicine.

Remember, the goal is to create cures that will have a long-term, positive impact on your body, making you healthier and boosting wellness. It's important to exercise caution when taking herbal medicines because it's possible to overdo them. Prescription and chemical treatment have a stronger effect, and doctors frequently prescribe particular doses to be taken.

Because herbal medicines take longer to work, you'll need to take them on a regular basis for a long time to observe results. Getting impatient and taking more will cause more harm than good. This is considered to be an abuse of herbal remedies and must be avoided at all costs. Anything done in excess is dangerous for us. People assume just because something is natural, it is safe, but that is not always the case.

It's easy to become overwhelmed by the sheer number of medicinal plants available, their various characteristics, and the several preparation methods that can be used. Herbs can be used for internal and external use. Some herbs you can eat, and others must be applied topically to the skin. Plant medicine is very powerful, so it's important to learn how to use it responsibly.

Internal Preparations

1. Decoction

What is an Herbal Decoction?

Herbal Decoction is an herbal preparation made by boiling herbs in a liquid, most commonly water. The reason for the decoction being made this way is that herbs have a lot of volatile oils within them, which extract during the boil. This is why when you boil an herb in water, its medicinal properties are released from the plant and into the water. When it is left to cool, it becomes a liquid with all its medicinal properties within it (Herbalismroots, 2016).

How to Make an Herbal Decoction

The most basic form of decoction is to boil the herbs in the water straight away to release any volatile oils within them. These volatile oils are the components that give herbs their medicinal properties. The volatile oils are extracted by boiling, and the water is discarded. The herbs are then gently simmered for some time. This is then strained and drunk immediately to avoid losing any medicinal properties.

The decoction can also be made with a slower process based on gentle simmering of the herbs in boiling water in an airtight container for some time. Then this is left to cool, and the remaining liquid is drunk (Mossy Meadow Farm, 2016).

Herbs to Use

So, which herbs make the best decoctions? It's truly a matter of taste, but keep in mind that the longer the herbs are allowed to simmer gently in the water, the stronger and more effective the decoction will be.

The following herbs are all good for making a decoction:

- Ashwagandha

- Cinnamon

- Dandelion root

- Chicory root

- Astragalus

- Mushrooms

- Milk thistle

- Rosehips

- Elderberries

- Ginger

Uses of Herbal Decoctions

- Used for diarrhea or dysentery.

- Also used for the treatment of kidney and liver problems.

- Decoctions can be mixed with other things like ginger which can help to further assist their effectiveness.

2. Infusions

What is an Herbal Infusion?

An herbal infusion is an herbal preparation that is made by steeping herbal ingredients in hot water. Herbs are able to absorb the water within the container, and their medicinal properties are released into it. As long as the container is kept cold, dry, and away from heat and light, the therapeutic characteristics will last for a long time.

How to Make Herbal Infusions

An herbal infusion is an herbal preparation made by steeping ingredients in hot water (Blog.mountainroseherbs, 2017).

The basic process is as follows:

- Soak the herbs in boiling water for about 15 minutes.

- Strain the liquid, squeeze out excess liquid and discard it.

- Rehydrate the herbs by putting them in a tea ball or something similar and making sure they are submerged under the liquid.

Herbs to Use

- Chamomile

- St. John's Wort

- Sage

- Peppermint

Uses of Herbal Infusions

- Easiest and most frequent way to prepare herbs for everyday use.

3. Tinctures

What are Herbal Tinctures?

A tincture is a herbal preparation produced by combining fresh or dried herbs with alcohol. The therapeutic components of the herb are extracted by the alcohol, which remains in the solution for a long time, depending on the amount of alcohol employed (Zen Maitri, 2016).

How to Make Herbal Tinctures

A tincture extracts the medicinal properties of herbs via alcohol. That same fluid alcohol will protect the medicine from degradation and damage. (Meagan, 2015).

Herbs to Use

- Chamomile

- Ginger

- Clove

Uses of Herbal Tinctures

- Used for insomnia and general anxiety relief.

4. Dry Preparations (Capsules or Tea)

What are Herbal Capsules?

An herbal is herbal ingredients encapsulated in gelatin which then can be injected into the body. This is the clinical alternative to using capsules that often come with pharmaceuticals or even certain foods. This way, you can avoid unnecessary additives and compounds that may have side effects and are not necessarily healthy for your body (JoybileeFarm 2016).

How to Make Herbal Capsules

Powdered herb is put into an appropriate size capsule and a small amount of water is added to make it pliable. The capsule is then filled with the mixture and rolled in order to ensure proper mixing. The capsules are then dried in the sun or placed in a dehydrator until they are completely dry.

How to Use Herbal Capsules

Herbal capsules can be taken orally, just like their pharmaceutical counterparts.

Herbs to Use

- Chamomile

- Ginger

Uses of Herbal Capsules

- Used to treat many issues, capsules can be helpful if taking an exact dose in a routine is important to your treatment.

5. Syrups

What is an Herbal Syrup?

An herbal syrup is a hybrid of honey and an herbal preparation. Honey is naturally sweet. However, if you make them by adding herbs to honey, the final product will possess a different flavor profile. In essence, the combination of honey and herb creates a natural sweetener.

How to Make an Herbal Syrup

An herbal syrup is a mixture of honey with herbal ingredients simmered and incorporated into it. It is made by combining the ingredients in a ratio that results in the right amount of sweetness in the final product.

How to Use Herbal Syrup

Herbal syrups are usually consumed as a sweetener. However, when they are cold, they can be used as a topical application in order to treat certain ailments (Meagan, 2015).

Herbs to Use

- Rosemary

Uses of Herbal Syrups

- Used in the treatment of ADD and ADHD.

- Can be used as a cooling agent or cough syrup for sore throat and colds.

The above preparations will last for the number of days listed below when used or stored properly.

- Decoctions—will last up to 3 days with proper storage.

- Infusions—will last up to 3 days with proper storage.

- Tinctures—will last up to 90 days with proper storage.

- Herbal Syrups—will last up to 4 weeks when stored properly. While there are no guaranteed shelf lives for herbs, given the fact that it's a mixture of honey and herbs, these preparations should be consumed within the three-week time frame for optimum freshness and efficacy.

External Use Preparations

1. Compresses

What is a Compress?

A compress is a topical application that has been soaked in an herbal preparation so that the medicinal properties are absorbed. This is then applied to the desired area in order to alleviate some of the ailments that may be present.

How to Make a Compress

To make a compress, you need:

- A clean container with a tight-fitting lid.

- An absorbent material like cotton or gauze.

- An herbal preparation that has been added to water.

- A way to heat up the container.

How to Use a Compress

- Take your desired herb and place it in a dry container.

- Fill the container up with hot water, and make sure that you do this slowly in order to not disturb the herbs or anything else located within it.

- Once the water has completely cooled, place the herbs in a tea ball or something similar so that they can be easily removed.

- Place it in the container, cover it with the lid and store it in a cool and dark place away from heat and light to preserve its properties.

Herbs to Use

- Chamomile

- St. John's Wort

- Lavender

Uses of Compress

- Used to treat inflammation, swelling, and allergic reactions in the affected area.

2. Salves

What is a Salve

A salve is a topical application that is used to treat many ailments like rashes, bruises, and insect bites. This external preparation works by having the active ingredients absorbed through your skin and into the bloodstream in order to bring about desired effects.

How to Make a Salve

To make a salve, you will need:

- An herb that has been dried.

- A way to mix the ingredients.

- A container to store the preparation in.

- An aluminum or stainless-steel bowl or something similar for the ingredients.

- Alcohol for storage purposes if desired.

- A blender or food processor.

- A set of measuring cups and spoons.

How to Use a Salve

- Take your dried herb and mix it up with the other ingredients in the bowl until you achieve the right consistency.

- Pour the salve into a smaller container like a jar and store it in a cool, dry area away from direct sunlight and heat.

Herbs to Use

- St. John's Wort

Uses of Salves

- Used as a pain reliever.

- Used to treat scars and burns.

- Can be used to treat insect bites.

- Can be used as an antiseptic.

3. Washes

What is a Wash?

A wash is a topical application that has been soaked in an herbal preparation so that the medicinal properties are absorbed. This is then applied to the desired area in order to alleviate some of the ailments that may be present.

How to Make a Wash

To make a wash, you will need:

- An herbal preparation that has been added to warm water.

- A clean container with a tight-fitting lid.

- An absorbent material like cotton or gauze.

- A way to heat up the container. If you're going to make this using water, add some boiling hot water after you've mixed everything together to activate the heat.

- Once the water is boiling hot, then you can use it. If you intend on using alcohol to make the wash, then you must heat it up in order to make sure that the alcohol has been activated.

How to Use a Wash

- Take your preferred herb and place it in a dry container.

- Fill the container with hot water, and make sure that you do this slowly in order to not disturb the herbs or anything else located within it.

- Once the water has completely cooled, place the herbs in a tea ball or something similar so that they can be easily removed.

- To keep its characteristics, place it in the container, cover it with the lid, and store it in a cold, dark area away from heat and light.

Herbs to Use

- Chamomile

- St. John's Wort

- Lavender

Uses of Washes

- Used in the treatment of wounds.

- Used for skincare and acne.

- Used for allergic reactions on the skin.

- Used as a mouthwash.

4. Poultice

What is a Poultice?

A poultice is an external preparation that contains herbs that have been made into a paste and are used to treat ailments like arthritis, swollen glands, and rashes by applying it to the desired area.

How to Make a Poultice

To make a poultice, you will need:

- An herbal preparation that has been made into a paste and is used as a paste.

- A way to mix ingredients up.

- A container for storage purposes if the poultice is being used for external application.

- Alcohol or some other preservative if you intend on storing the preparation for an extended period of time.

- An aluminum or stainless-steel bowl for the ingredients. You'll need special equipment if you're using a food processor for this.

- Clean cloth to apply the paste.

How to Use a Poultice

- Wrap the clean cloth around your hand and apply the paste to the affected area in order for it to be absorbed through your skin.

Herbs to Use

- St. John's Wort

Uses of Poultice

- Used to treat arthritis and other pains as well as wounds

- Can be used for the treatment of earaches and sore throats by applying it externally to the afflicted area

- It can be used on scabies or mites in order to prevent them from becoming infected (Meagan, 2015)

The above preparations will last for the number of days listed below when used and stored properly

- Compress - will last up to 10 days

- Salve - can be stored for 6-8 months

- Wash - can be stored for 2 weeks if it has been powered with alcohol, you can store it for up to 4 weeks if it is not powered with alcohol

- Poultice - can be stored for 1-2 days

Chapter Six:
Step 5 - Identify What You Need

Now that you have gone through the steps of making your herbal remedies, the next thing is to identify the correct treatment that you want to use. In our HEALING framework, the letter "I" stands for *"Identify What You Need."*

As much as you enjoy a well-stocked herbal medicine cabinet, some remedies are best prepared when you're about to use them, while some have shorter shelf lives. Plus, you may not have enough space to cover every possible health concern. That's why it's essential to identify what types of remedies you need so you know exactly what it is you need to buy and prepare.

Millions of people in the United States are misdiagnosed every year with diseases they don't have. Approximately half of these misdiagnoses result in serious harm.

A person's health can be jeopardized by a misdiagnosis. They can cause delays in recovery and occasionally necessitate dangerous therapy. An estimated 40 thousand patients who enter intensive care units die due to a misdiagnosis each year.

In 2016, Healthline released an article highlighting the dangers of misdiagnoses and how misdiagnoses affected the lives of three people with three distinct health issues.

A 14-year-old girl named Nina was also among the victims. As a result, cramps, an eating disorder, and mental health issues were misdiagnosed. Endometriosis is a serious condition that affects a person's reproductive organs. The doctors even suggested she had been abused as a child, which was the reason she acted out. Her friends at school made her a laughing stock for being "sensitive." It took 11 years of misdiagnosis before she was finally diagnosed. Right before her 25th birthday, her gynecologist performed a laparoscopic surgery, which was successful.

Her story is a testament to how misdiagnosis can cause serious health issues and can also affect a person's overall well-being. Many people misdiagnose a host of conditions; some are lucky enough to get the symptoms of their diseases under control before they are set a course of treatment. Others are not (Healthline, 2016). In this chapter, we'll talk about some of the go-tos to stock up on in terms of herbs, as well as the usual ailments that can be resolved with natural medicine.

Identifying the extent of your health and then knowing the quality and quantity of what you need can help boost your self-esteem and confidence. The more herbs and remedies you have, the more likely they are to heal your ailments.

To make things easier, we'll also provide suggestions on how to identify your ailments so you can decide which herbal medicine is most effective for you.

1. Pain Relief

Herbs that can help

- Lavender

What it can help with: Muscle aches and pains. Tension headaches.

Consume through inhalation or topically.

Precautions: Generally safe if used properly.

2. Allergies

Herbs that can help

- Echinacea

What it can help with: Treating both the symptoms and the root cause of allergies.

Consume topically and as a supplement.

Precautions: May cause side effects for people who have epilepsy or convulsions or who are pregnant or breastfeeding.

3. Colds and Flu

Herbs that Can Help

- Elderberry

What it can help with: Treating colds and flu.

Consume through inhalation, as a syrup or as a supplement.

Precautions: If consumed in large amounts, they may cause some side effects, including nausea, vomiting, abdominal pain, and diarrhea.

4. Heartburn and Indigestion

Herbs that can help

- Chamomile

What it can help with: Heartburn, indigestion, upset stomach.

Consume topically and as a supplement.

Precautions: May cause some side effects such as diarrhea and vomiting.

5. Antiviral and Antibacterial

Herbs that can help

- Garlic

What it can help with: Treatment of viruses and infections

Consume topically or as a supplement

Precautions: May cause side effects like cramping, nausea, and diarrhea.

6. Mental Health Concerns

Herbs that can help

- St. John's Wort

What it can help with: Treating depression, improving mood and anxiety.

Consume topically or as a supplement.

Precautions: Has the potential to cause birth defects, so use at your own risk.

7. Headaches

Herbs that can help

- Peppermint

What it can help with: Treating headaches.

Consume through inhalation or as a supplement.

Precautions: May cause some side effects like diarrhea, cramping, and nausea.

8. Wounds and Burns

Herbs that can help

- Chamomile

- Aloe

- Gotu kola

What it can help with: Treating wounds, burns, and ulcers.

Consume topically or as a supplement.

Precautions: May cause some side effects like itching, burning, and flaking (St. Luke's Hospital, 2016).

9. Insect Bites & Stings

Herbs that can help

- Basil

- Echinacea

- Peppermint

What it can help with: Treating insect bites and stings.

Consume through inhalation or as a supplement.

Precautions: May cause some side effects like itching, redness, and swelling (Wishgardenherbs, 2018).

What Are the Most Effective Natural Antibiotics?

Do you know what the most effective natural antibiotics are? Many people are under the impression that natural antibiotics are not as effective as those produced with pharmaceuticals. For this reason, it is important to understand the role that these herbs play when it comes to fighting infection.

Many people know about certain plant extracts that can be used for treatment and prevention but are not necessarily aware of the role natural antibiotics can play in boosting their immune system and preventing infections. Folk remedies have been used for generations for medicinal purposes, including extracts from plants, roots, seeds, and fruits. Natural antibiotics can promote a well-balanced immune system with the help of herbs that fight bacterial infections.

When it comes to health, many people want to make changes and begin incorporating natural, herbal remedies with the hope of restoring balance and finding relief from chronic ailments that haven't responded to conventional medical treatment.

In fact, no matter how good your current prescription medications are, you will always have a lot of options to choose from if you are looking for natural alternatives. Certain herbs can be taken into your system and work together with the medication you are presently taking. Unfortunately, many people do not realize the potential benefits that they can enjoy when they use natural herbal medicine (Chaunie Brusie, 2019).

The following are the most effective natural antibiotics that you should rely on for common infectious agents:

Garlic Extract

For many years, garlic has been used to treat a variety of conditions. It is one of the most effective natural antibiotics that you can use as part of your daily regimen to ward off infections and boost your immune system.

Thyme Essential Oil

This natural antibiotic is frequently used to treat both upper respiratory infections, acute infections, and chronic sinusitis. It works to fight bacteria and viruses, including the common cold.

Oregano Oil

Oregano oil is derived from basil and offers a high concentration of carvacrol. This natural antibiotic has been found to work well in the treatment of oral, gastrointestinal, and urinary tract infections.

Honey

This natural antibiotic is a powerhouse that helps to fight infection by producing hydrogen peroxide, and it works to destroy various microorganisms like streptococcus and staphylococcus.

Myrrh Extract

This natural antibiotic is often used to treat sore throats and colds, ear infections, and other disorders. Myrrh has a high concentration of thymol, tannins as well as thymic acid that fights infections.

Echinacea

This natural antibiotic is derived from the purple coneflower plant. It has been used since the beginning of time to treat diseases and illnesses ranging in severity.

Cloves

Cloves have been used in the Middle East to treat dental problems, mouth and gum inflammation, chronic coughs, as well as toothaches. This natural antibiotic has been found to reduce the impact of oral bacteria.

Creating Your Own Herbal First Aid Kit

Many people have become more interested in herbal medicine because of their desire to find effective natural antibiotics. Many are taking the time to learn about different herbs, so they can formulate their own first aid kit with the herbs that they feel could benefit them the most.

Patients who take supplements and those who like to rely on herbal medicine will understand why it is important to create your own first aid kit, so you will be able to treat minor ailments quickly with the help of natural remedies that heal you from within.

The 3 types of herbal first aid kits that you can create:

1. Herbal First Aid Kit: A Must-Have for Your Home

Creating your own herbal first aid kit is a must. Not only is it necessary to have the items on hand, you will also need to know how to use them. This is where doing some research on common herbs and ailments helps. Once you have gathered all the necessary items, you may want to keep a notebook on hand with a list of common herbs and ailments as well as their medicinal properties.

2. Herbal First Aid Kits: Everyday Carry

Many people like to enjoy their active lifestyles and plan on spending time outdoors. That is why it is important to have a herbal first aid kit that you can take with you wherever you go. This way, you will always have a good supply of herbs and remedies with you at all times.

3. Herbal Field Kit/Evacuation Kit

You will want to research what supplies you will need for the evacuation of your home or workplace. Consider the possibility that you may have mold or asbestos in your area, and you must have a safe place to go until the danger has passed.

Herbs and other natural remedies can help to restore balance in your immune system. It is important that you find what works best for you so that you can improve your overall health and wellness (Dickinson, 2016).

Choosing The Right Herbal Remedies for You

There are countless herbal remedies available on the market, and you may be a bit overwhelmed.

Here are a few things you should keep in mind when choosing your herbal remedies:

1. Figure Out What Support You Need

Looking at your own body and lifestyle will help you to determine what type of remedies will work best for you. Do you need a supplement that will boost your immune system? A natural antibiotic that is going to fight infection? Or perhaps you would like another type of medicine to treat your symptoms.

2. What To Incorporate Into Your Routine?

Figure out what you can actually take on a daily basis. The format, time, and ways to incorporate herbs into your daily routine are vital considerations.

3. Do Your Own Research

It has to be stressed that you must always do your research. It is important to understand the constituents and how they will help your body to get better. Researching which herbs or supplements suit your situation is a must.

4. Consider Other Ways to Add Plants to Your Life

Find out which other herbs and plants you can use in your daily life. There are many ways to be more holistic, like adding different types of plants to your diet.

5. Geography And Heritage

Keep in mind that there are different herbs in different regions. Some have been used for a long time by specific races or ethnic groups. Remembering this will help you to know what to look for and how to obtain them (Robinett, 2021).

CHAPTER SEVEN:
STEP 6 - NOW START CONCOCTING!

Now comes the most fun part: creating your remedies. You'll feel like a mad scientist or a witch creating a magic potion. "N' is the next letter in our acronym, HEALING framework, and it stands for "Now Start Concocting."

In this chapter, we will explore all the things you can do to create your own herbal remedy for the ailments discussed in chapter 5.

Using natural remedies as alternative or primary treatments is a very important aspect of alternative medicine. Natural remedies offer many advantages over standard pharmaceuticals, and you may find yourself saving a considerable sum of money, too.

Would you use a drug if it could be made from a particular herb? Would you use it if you could pick it right off the bush at the roadside? Some may say no because herbs are not a drug, they are not synthetically made in a lab. However, you can use them safely and effectively to address your ailments without the fear of overdosing or becoming ill from an adverse reaction. Natural remedies allow you to have more control over your health. According to estimates, up to 36% of US citizens aged 18 and up utilize complementary and alternative medicine.

More and more people are paying attention to herbal treatment, but not all of them are happy with their current results. Some say that it is hard for them to decipher what herbs actually work for what ailment. People are also concerned about the potential side effects of herbal remedies.

Understanding and choosing the right natural remedies is not an easy task. Some people have turned to herbal supplements or tinctures, which they can buy in health food stores or supermarkets.

When you're just getting started, it's best to buy ready-made herbal supplements from reputable suppliers or build your own from scratch using a recipe. This can help you begin to learn about herbal remedies and gain experience in their use.

In your arsenal, you should own many herbs. Not all herbal remedies are created equal, and some can be more effective than others. You should have at least ten to twenty common herbs on hand so you can make several remedies that will be effective for a variety of symptoms.

When you use herbal remedies, know the difference between herbs that have been crushed and ones that have been made into tinctures. When making your own remedies, you can add the herb to a liquid in a glass bottle for administering it orally. The other option is to add it to a capsule or an oil.

You'll find recipes and instructions for making your own herbal medicine in this chapter.

There are many ways to make remedies. You can use an alcohol burner for preparing a tincture or a liquid extract, both of which are methods of adding herbs to water. You can also opt for an herbal tea or a traditional herbal remedy that is just made from raw herbs and water.

Whichever you choose, be sure to read the recipe carefully and follow it exactly the way it was written. Don't add too much of anything. Herbs are potent and should not be used in excess.

PAIN RELIEF

Greaseless Pain Ointment

Indications: Say goodbye to aches, pains, sprains, strains, and bruises with this herbal pain ointment. Apply it several times a day for the best results.

Ingredients:

- Coconut oil (25 grams)

- Infused oil, arnica + St. John's wort (3/4 cup)

- Helichrysum hydrosol (2/3 cup)

- Shea butter (20 grams)

- Lavender essential oil (40 drops)

- Beeswax (20 grams)

Directions:

1. Place the beeswax, coconut oil, and shea butter in your double boiler. Heat the mixture on low to allow the ingredients to melt.

2. Once completely melted, top the mixture with the arnica and St. John's wort-infused oil. Use a popsicle stick to stir everything as you go.

3. Once the beeswax starts to solidify, turn off the double boiler. Stir the mixture again to make sure everything is well-combined. You may reheat the mixture to ensure that the beeswax is completely melted.

4. Pour the melted, still-warm ointment mixture into a food processor or blender. Let the mixture sit until it has adequately cooled and becomes semi-solid.

5. Turn the food processor or blender on before gradually trickling in the coconut oil, lavender essential oil, and helichrysum hydrosol. Stir everything as you go.

6. Before the ointment completely solidifies, transfer it into a glass container and store it in a cool place.

Meadowsweet Pain Elixir

Indications: This elixir is safe for most individuals, although you may have to use it with caution if you have the flu, chickenpox, or asthma.

Ingredients:

- Meadowsweet flowers (100 grams)

- Glycerin (100 milliliters)

- Vodka, 50-% (400 milliliters)

Directions:

1. Take a large glass jar and fill it with the meadowsweet flowers.

2. Pour the glycerin and vodka into the jar. Shake well to combine everything.

3. Let the mixture stand for one month to six weeks. To ensure that the meadowsweet flowers stay covered by a liquid, weigh them down with a weight or a clean stone. You may also add more alcohol to cover the flowers, which gradually absorb the liquid.

4. Pour the mixture through a clean cheesecloth.

5. Transfer the strained mixture into a labeled bottle.

Ginger Fomentation

Indications: Muscle spasms and menstrual cramps can be eased by this easy-to-make ginger fomentation.

Ingredients:

- Water (2 cups)

- Cramp bark (1/4 cup)

- Ginger, dried (1/4 cup)

- Cayenne powder (1 tablespoon)

Directions:

1. Fill a pan with the water before adding the cayenne powder and cramp bark.

2. Cover the pan and heat on medium, let simmer for about twenty to thirty minutes.

3. Strain the mixture, and then let it stand until it is warm to the touch.

4. To use your ginger fomentation, dip a clean washcloth in it. Wring out any excess liquid from the cloth, then place it on your affected area. Top the cloth with your hot water bottle before covering it with a towel. Allow the fomentation to do its work for about twenty minutes to one hour.

COLDS AND FLU

Chamomile Herbal Steam

Indications: Relieving a stuffy nose is not a problem with this effective stuffy nose remedy. (You may reuse this chamomile tea several times, after which you can use it in your garden for composting.)

Ingredients:

- Chamomile flowers, dried (2 handfuls)

- Water (2 quarts)

Directions:

1. Pour the water into a pot and heat on medium-high. Allow the water to boil before turning off the heat and adding the dried chamomile flowers.

2. Cover the pot and allow the mixture to boil for an additional fifteen minutes.

3. Remove the pot from the heat and let stand on a large hot pad.

4. With plenty of tissues as well as a large towel on hand, remove the pot cover.

5. Holding your face over the steaming pot, place the towel on top of your head. Breathe in through the nose and mouth to let the steam unclog your stuffy nose

(use the tissues to wipe your nose). Do this for five to fifteen minutes or until your stuffy nose is relieved.

Herbal Colds And Flu Tincture

Indications: This spicy tincture, also known as 'fire cider', has antibiotic and antiseptic properties that make it effective as a cold and flu herbal remedy. Take 1 teaspoon per hour when a cold or flu acts up.

Ingredients:

- Vinegar, White or Apple Cider (1 cup)

- Horseradish, fresh, grated (1 ½ tablespoon)

- Ginger, fresh, grated (1 ½ tablespoon)

- Onion, minced (½ cup)

- Garlic, minced (1 ½ tablespoon)

- Honey (1/3 cup)

- Mustard seeds (1 ½ tablespoon)

- Black peppercorns (1 ½ tablespoon)

- Cayenne chilies, whole (1 to 2 pieces) or chili flakes, dried (1 teaspoon)

Directions:

1. Take a glass jar (1 pint) and fill it with the minced garlic and onion.

2. Add the grated horseradish and ginger along with the peppercorns, whole cayenne chilies or dried chili flakes, and mustard seeds. Stir well to combine.

3. Top the mixture with the vinegar, making sure there is an inch of liquid above the rest of the ingredients.

4. Cover with a lid made of plastic material. Allow the mixture to sit for two weeks, shaking the jar every day to ensure that the liquid and herbs are mixed.

5. Use a clean cheesecloth to strain the mixture.

6. Add the honey into the mixture before pouring it into a clean, labeled bottle and storing it in the cupboard.

HEARTBURN AND INDIGESTION

Marshmallow Root Pastilles

Indications: These cooling, soothing marshmallow root pastilles work effectively in treating sore throats as well as heartburn, ulcers, and other digestive problems.

Ingredients:

- Rose petals, powdered (1 tablespoon)

- Sage leaves, powdered (1/2 tablespoon)

- Marshmallow root (2 tablespoons)

- Honey, raw, warmed (1 ½ tablespoon)

- Cinnamon powder (1/2 tablespoon)

- Rose powder (1/2 tablespoon)

Directions:

1. Combine the marshmallow root with powdered rose petals and sage leaves in a mixing bowl.

2. Meanwhile, warm the honey in a small saucepan heated on medium. Make sure it never gets too hot, but just warm enough to have the consistency of a syrup.

3. Once the honey is warm, pour it into the herb mixture in small amounts, stirring as you go. Keep stirring until you end up with a soft dough that is just sticky enough.

4. Use your clean hands to mold the pastille dough into small balls.

5. Sprinkle cinnamon and rose petal powders on the prepared pastilles before using immediately or storing them in the refrigerator for about two weeks.

Chamomile–Angelica Tea

Ingredients:

- 2 cups of boiling water

- 2 tsp. dried angelica

- 1 ½ tsp. dried chamomile

Utensils Needed:

- 1 large mug

- A kettle

Instructions:

1. Boil 2 cups of water.

2. Pour it into a large mug and add the dried herbs.

3. Let it steep for 15 minutes and strain. Serve and sip gently.

4. Take your time to enjoy the refreshing tastes.

5. Take this 5–6 times daily.

Advice:

- Not to be taken by pregnant women.

- If you're allergic to ragweed, please do not take it.

Ginger Syrup

Ingredients:

- 3 oz. fresh ginger root, chopped

- 3 cups water

- 1 ½ cups honey

Instructions:

1. Combine ginger and water in a saucepan, then boil over low heat until water is reduced to half.

2. Pour the content into a measuring cup and back into a new saucepan through the cheesecloth to sieve the liquid. Wring the cheesecloth until no water is left.

3. Add honey to the mixture and heat it again on low heat. Mix thoroughly together.

4. Then, pour the syrup into a bottle and refrigerate. Label it.

5. Shake well and take just 2 tbsps, 4 times daily whenever you want to use it.

Advice:

- Younger children under the age of 13 should take just 2 times per day. Not for children under 1-year-old.

- If you're on any blood-thinning medication, try as much as possible to avoid this herbal medicine.

- Do not use this remedy if you have any internal disease like gallbladder disease or a bleeding disorder.

HEADACHES

Cooling Headache Tea

Ingredients:

- 2 tablespoons fresh mint leaves, roughly chopped

- 1 tablespoon fresh thyme leaves, finely chopped

- 1 teaspoon anise seeds, crush in a mortar, or zest from a lemon in a spice grinder

- 5 cups boiling water

Instructions:

1. Boil 5 cups of water, pour over the herbs, and let steep for 5 minutes before straining into a jug.

2. Pour into mugs and drink while hot or let it cool down and add ice cubes for a refreshing cold version.

Warming Headache Tea

Ingredients:

- 1 tablespoon cinnamon

- 2 cloves

- 1 tablespoon ginger

- 1 tablespoon cayenne pepper flakes

- 2 teabags

- water (about 2 cups)

Directions:

1. Add about 4 tablespoons of water to a small pot and bring it to a boil.

2. Add the tea bags filled with spices and cayenne pepper flakes and allow boiling for about 5 minutes straight. Remove from heat just before the tea turns black or becomes bitter.

3. Allow the tea to cool slightly before drinking it. Add honey for sweetness if desired. Drink once a day until symptoms disappear or on an as-needed basis if pain persists after relieving symptoms.

Peppery Headache Tea

Ingredients:

- 1 tablespoon ginger

- 1 teaspoon dried pepper pods

- 1-liter of water

Instructions:

1. Bring the water to a boil. Make sure to turn the heat off,

2. Add ginger and pepper, and

3. Steep covered for 5 minutes.

4. Strain and enjoy

ALLERGIES

Feverfew-Peppermint Tincture

During an allergic attack, feverfew or peppermint clear up the airways. If you don't have feverfew, prepare this tincture using just peppermint. The tincture will last up to 7 years in a cold, dark location.

Ingredients:

- 6 oz dried peppermint

- 2 oz dried feverfew

- 2 cups vodka, 80 proof, unflavored

Directions:

1. Combine the feverfew or peppermint in a sterilized pint jar. Fill the jar to the top with vodka.

2. Tightly close the jar and give it a good shake. For 6 to 8 weeks, keep it in a cold, dark cabinet and shake it many times a week.

3. Soak a sheet of cheesecloth in water and lay it over the funnel's mouth. Pour the tincture into another sterilized pint jar using the funnel. Remove the moisture from the herbs by wringing them out. Transfer the completed medicine to dark-colored glass bottles after discarding the wasted herbs.

4. When allergy symptoms flare up, use five drops orally. If the flavor is too intense for you, combine it with some water or juice to consume it.

Caution:

If you are sensitive to ragweed, do not take feverfew. It should not be used during pregnancy.

WOUNDS, CUTS, SCRAPES

Goldenseal and Sumac

This treatment significantly helps with pains and helps heal faster for internal and external wounds.

Ingredients:

- 1 tsp. dried goldenseal leaves

- 1 tsp. dried sumac leaves

- 3 tbsps. hot water

Instructions:

1. Use a grinder to grind the herbs into a soft powder, then enclose them in a small, thick infuser pack.

2. Boil the pack in some water for not more than 5 minutes. Remove from water and let it cool so as not to burn yourself.

3. Put a very light cloth on the sore. Place the packet over the sore and leave for about 20 minutes.

4. Repeat this 2-3 times daily.

Topical Application for Abrasions

Ingredients:

- 1teaspoon of white pine inner bark

- 1 teaspoon of wild cherry bark

- 1teaspoon of wild plum root

Instructions:

1. Boil until the bark and roots are soft.

2. Cool and strain.

3. To use, soak a clean (preferably sterilized) cloth in the solution and apply it to the affected area.

Wound Wash

When cleaning, try a simple toner with rose water or witch hazel extract if you're in a hurry. Then you can use a formula like this for soaks and compressions. You might consider adding ½ cup dried marshmallow or kelp for emollient effects as the wound heals.

Ingredients:

- ½ cup dried calendula flower

- ½ cup dried plantain leaf

- ½ cup dried rose petals

- ½ cup dried goldenrod leaf and flower

- ¼ cup dried chamomile flower

- ¼ cup dried self-heal leaf and flower

- ¼ cup dried St. John's wort leaf and flower

- ¼ cup dried yarrow leaf and flower

- Salt, for the infusion

- 1 cup boiling water

Instructions:

1. Mix all the herbs. Store in an airtight container.

2. When needed, take 1-2 tablespoons of herb mix, and place it in boiling water. Steep for 15 minutes, then strain.

3. Stir in 1 teaspoon of salt for each quart of infusion you've made.

4. Let it cool.

5. Soak the wounded part or apply a compress over the affected area.

6. Repeat as frequently as you can, at least three times per day.

BURNS

Healing Honey

Honey is one of the best healing agents for burns: If you have nothing to compare or get some other options, plain honey is still an excellent remedy on its own. It gets even better, though, when you try to infuse all these healing herbs into it ahead of time.

Ingredients:

- ½ cup fresh calendula flower

- ½ cup fresh rose petals

- 1-tbsp honey, gently warmed

Instructions:

1. Put the calendula and rose petals in a pint-size mason jar.

2. Fill the jar with warm honey. Seal the jar and place it in a warm area to infuse for 1 month.

3. Use a double boiler to gently warm the closed jar in water until the honey gets a liquid consistency. Next, strain all the infused honey into a new jar, pressing against the strainer to extract as much honey as you can.

4. After cleaning a burn site, apply a layer of the infused honey and then cover lightly with a gauze bandage. Refresh all the applications at least twice a day.

Fresh Aloe Vera Gel

Eases sunburn pain, mild burns, and psoriasis.

Aloe is a very common ingredient in sunburn ointments. In its natural state, it helps heal and moisturize the skin. It helps with any skin issue involving redness and itchiness.

Ingredients:

- Aloe Vera plant

Tools Needed:

- Knife

- Cotton

Instructions:

1. Cut 2 inches from the aloe vera leaf.

2. Use a sharp knife to cut out the tip, use cotton to take some gel, and apply generously on the burn.

3. Do this 3-4 times daily.

BITES AND STINGS

Cooling Compress

The cooling sensation peppermint provides to the skin is attributed to its menthol content as well as its ability to increase blood circulation and disperse irritants from bites and stings.

Ingredients:

- 16 fluid ounces of water

- ½ cup dried peppermint leaf

- ¼ cup Epsom salts

Instructions:

1. Combine all the ingredients. Cover and bring to a boil. Remove from the heat.

2. Using a cloth, soak it in the mixture. Strain a bit and apply the cloth to the bite or sting.

IMMUNITY BOOSTING

Cleansing Aloe Water

Used for: Detoxing, constipation relief, heartburn relief.

This aloe water can help with stomach issues like constipation.

People also drink aloe water to boost their energy and immunity. If you haven't eaten aloe before, we recommend talking to a professional first.

Only ingest a small amount at a time as aloe can have laxative effects.

Ingredients:

- ½-teaspoon or 1 tablespoon aloe gel

- 1 cup water

Directions:

1. Scrape out gel from a fresh-cut leaf into a blender or food processor. If you have never ingested aloe before, start with just ½ teaspoon.

2. Blend with water and drink!

3. To make the beverage tastier, you can add other ingredients like 100% fruit juice, cucumber, parsley, or raw honey.

SKINCARE

Honey and Milk Mask

Ingredients:

- 1 tsp. honey

- 3 tsp. milk

- ½ cucumber

- 5 drops of fresh-squeezed lemon juice

Directions:

Mix all the ingredients thoroughly and gently massage the mask onto your face with fingers. Leave on for 15 minutes, then rinse off with water.

Firming Face Mask

Ingredients:

- 2 egg whites separated from the yolk

- 1 tbsp yogurt

Directions:

Mix yogurt and eggs. Wash your face with warm water after leaving on the mask for 10 minutes.

Honey and Clay Mask

Ingredients:

- 1 tbsp. white clay

- 1 tbsp. honey

- 1 tsp. warm water

- 1 tsp. olive oil

Directions:

1. Mix clay and honey with a little warm water.

2. Add olive oil and stir.

3. Apply to face

4. Wash off after 20 minutes with cold water.

White Clay Mask

Ingredients:

- 2 tbsp. oats

- 1 tbsp. white clay

- 3-4 tbsp. milk

Directions:

1. Boil the oatmeal,

2. Allow to cool

3. Mix it with 1 tablespoon of clay and 3-4 tablespoons of milk

4. Apply mask to face

5. Rinse off with warm water after 20 minutes

Lifting Honey and Clay Mask

Ingredients:

- 1 tbsp honey

- 2 tbsp lemon juice

- 1 tbsp white clay

Directions:

1. Mix ingredients well and

2. Apply the mixture to your skin using your fingers.

3. Cover your face with a thin, even layer

4. Allow to dry for 15 minutes

5. Wash with cool water

Anti-aging Red Wine Face Mask

Ingredients:

- 1 egg white

- 2 tbsp. red wine

- 1 tbsp. honey

Directions:

1. Mix the egg white, red wine, and honey until you have a smooth substance

2. Spread the paste with your fingertips on your clean face and neck, avoiding the eye area.

3. Leave the mask on for 10-15 minutes,

4. Wash it off with lukewarm water.

Chapter Eight:
Step 7 - Get Comfortable with Formulation

Part of getting better at herbalism is learning not just to follow a recipe but learning to formulate your own herbal recipes based on your specific needs, requirements, and preferences.

In this chapter, you will learn about the letter "G" in our herbal medicine HEALING framework, meaning "Get Comfortable with Formulation."

The Letter "G" is all about getting excited about formula creation, getting comfortable with making many formulations, experimenting with your favorite formulas, and learning which ones work best for you.

It is similar to the creative process you would use when creating original artwork.

Or think of it as a fun project in chemistry. You will be "playing" with your formula components to discover new recipes and to determine which ingredients work best for your specific needs.

Product personalization has become a big trend within the health and beauty industry. With this in mind, you can use your herbalism to personalize your product line.

Often, you will find that the process of formula creation is a highly educational experience for you. When you discover something new about a formula or when it works better than expected, it will reinforce your understanding of herbs and nourish your herbal connections.

By trying out many components and combinations of them in your formulas, you will learn which ones help with specific situations more than others. If you have a formula that seems to be working very well, you may want to make larger quantities of it and keep it on hand as a basic go-to recipe.

By carefully studying herbal plants and their actions, you will discover which herbs work best for specific situations. You will also learn which herbs work well together in formulas. The more attention that you give to the details, the better your herbalism will become over time.

Customers desire personalization, and businesses are responding by providing it. Having something specifically tailored to you is so desirable for many.

When products are tailor-made to suit an individual's needs, they can save money and time because they don't have to purchase or make large quantities or inventories of products that may not be needed. For example, a customer with allergies does not have to worry about ingredients that could cause an allergic reaction.

The second reason is convenience. As consumers, we are always looking for something convenient and easy to use. We want things that can be customized and tailored to our exact needs. The third reason is that personalization creates a relationship. When customers feel like a company cares about them and their needs, they are more likely to seek the company out in the future if they need more of those same products.

This is just as true in the herbalism world. When people buy herbal products, they want to know that their needs are unique and that their purchase has been crafted specifically for them.

When you learn to build your herbal formulas, you will be able to satisfy this need. As a result, you may see larger numbers of repeat sales from your regular customers.

The flip side of personalization is the fact that few people can create effective formulas on their own. Some people have strong interests in herbalism and want to take this route, but many do not.

The NY Times article talks about pharmaceuticals being able to adjust ingredients based on a patient's age, gender, weight, genetic factors, and previous responses to different dosage levels. This is the same type of customization that is available in the herbal industry. Many people want to take the herbal route but don't know where to start.

There are many ways that you can make personalized products for your customers, and with more knowledge about herbs and their actions, you will develop a formula that works for them.

The Art of Formulation

Creating simple herbal formulas is a simple process, and you will find that the more you practice, the better you become. There are no hard and fast rules when it comes to herbal formulas, though. The best formulas are always made with what works for each patient.

As you continue to do your research, experimenting together with your patients as well as with herbs, you will get a better understanding of what works for each person. This is where the fun begins in herbalism.

Including herbs that work well together or herbs that activate specific actions of other herbs can lead to successful formula creation. Using spices and extracts to create herbal formulas is common these days, and they are an easy way to add flavor and aroma. You can also use spices and extracts in conjunction with beeswax products, which have a strong natural aromatic quality.

You will learn through this book how important it is to be creative with your formulas so that you can find what works best for you.

Simpling vs. Formulating

A simple herb remedy is made up of a single herb. One of the most common reasons for creating a simple preparation is to use it with children or pets, who often cannot tolerate tinctures or teas.

The other reason for making simple preparations is that it can be easier to create more rather than less. Once you understand which herbs are most effective, it becomes easier and faster to come up with many different formulas. Creating simples is the best way to become familiar with the recognized actions of herbs so that you can combine them in future recipes.

In contrast, a complex formula consists of multiple herbs. The simplest type of complex formula is one that contains just two herbs. Herbal formulas are very flexible, and you will find that they work in many ways.

There are some cases where it is easier to create a simple formula using a single herb as the main ingredient. When you have multiple herbs, adding an extra herb to the formulation can make them more effective and can improve their potency.

When you combine herbs, you have a synergy of herbs, meaning that their actions are more powerful than if they were used individually. When you use both herbs well, you will get the best results because each herb has already been tested and added to your formula.

This can be very helpful when a patient's needs change over time, and the formula needs to be adjusted to meet those new needs. When you make simple formulas, this is not an issue, but as you make complex formulas, it's something that can come into play.

Formulating Your Own Herbal Remedies

There are many types of formulas, and you can customize each one to meet the specific needs of your customers. The best way to be successful with herbal formulas is by being creative.

As you begin looking over the herbs in this book, you will recognize what might work well together and which herbs are easier to use and create simples and formulas with.

Working with your customers, who all have different needs, will provide you with more understanding as to what they need.

Following a simple recipe is a good way to get you started. Recipes help you get familiar with the different ingredients, equipment, and measurements used in herbal remedies. It is also an easy way to understand the use of each ingredient, like which emulsifier to use in which product.

You can follow a set recipe and then change a few ingredients to make it your recipe. However, when you copy a recipe without learning about the science behind each ingredient and how it interacts with other components, you won't be able to learn how to create your formula. You'll be only imitating a recipe with all its mistakes and not knowing how to fix it when it doesn't work for your body as you expected.

Recipes also mean you can only produce things that other people share online. You can't create your products without learning about the correct percentage of each ingredient and which items go together. If you make a mistake, you may have an unsafe product on your hands, and you won't know it unless you try it on yourself, which can be extremely harmful.

On the other hand, using formulas to create your products involves knowledge and practice of all the possible ingredients you can use. It is how you can learn to make a safe and effective product designed for a specific purpose. Formulations will teach you how to create a product from scratch, unlike recipes another person creates.

A formula will tell you how to alter a specific ingredient. You'll keep experimenting with different batches until you reach the desired results. While a *recipe* includes measurements like tablespoons, liters, or fluid ounces, a *formula* involves a specific percentage of each item.

Volume measurements in recipes cannot be accurate when replicated on a large scale. This is because they are subject to alteration due to temperature changes. You need to ensure that each batch has the right texture, odor, and effectiveness. This is why it is important to switch to a formula, especially when creating a large batch.

Why Formulas Are Better than Recipes

You can create a mass production line when you follow a specific formula. Each ingredient is weighed in grams or pounds before its amount can be calculated in each product.

Having a formula with a percentage can indicate which item to increase or decrease during your experimentation phase.

Suppose you're making a moisturizing cream for dry skin. In that case, you can increase the percentage of certain oils (say from 40% to 60%) while decreasing the number of other ingredients (say from 60% to 40%) to end up with a 100% formula in total. A percentage is also an indicator of the safe amount of each ingredient.

The science behind formulas will also teach you how to substitute ingredients. When some items are not available, you can replace them with others with the same effects. This knowledge gives you many options to choose from and helps you to keep the production line going.

If you just follow someone's recipe, you may not be able to make necessary alterations or improve your products because you won't understand the effect of each ingredient in certain amounts. You'll keep trying to change a few things here and there to identify the problems with your product and, in the process, waste a lot of time and effort, not to mention money as well.

On the other hand, creating a formula gives you the advantage of having the basics to create a high-quality product. By studying the core functions of each active constituent, you'll be able to understand what works for your body and constitution. You can build on this knowledge for future products!

How to Create a Standard Formula

When creating a standard formula for any product, there are specific requirements that you need to include. Suppose you're creating a skincare product like a facial moisturizer. In that case, a standard formula is used to explain the ingredients in a universal unit: *the percentage by weight.* This means it can be followed and understood globally because some countries use the metric system and others use the imperial system.

A percentage shows you the safe levels of each ingredient. For example, moisturizers should not have a percentage of essential oils that exceeds 1%. If this information was written in drops or volume measurements, it could become confusing and require a prolonged calculation. This is why a formula is a proper method for mapping out all the ingredients in a product.

You can use a formula to make personal or manufacturing-grade batches. It is also easier to alter the percentage of each ingredient. For example, suppose your cream is too runny. In that case, you can increase the percentage of beeswax to make it firmer and decrease the percentage of another ingredient like carrier oil. A standard formula is a requirement when you register your product if you're aiming to sell your brand.

Here's a list of all the requirements that must be written in a standard formula for cosmetic and medicinal products:

1. Each ingredient must be written next to its percentage by weight. The formula must be written to reach a

total of 100%. It is inaccurate to write the formula to reach a specific number of bottles as follows: "This formula is for 100 jars." All volume and weight measurements in ml, g, drops, teaspoons, tablespoons, and so forth should be converted to a percentage by weight. This step is helpful because you can use this percentage to calculate any number of jars or bottles and get an accurate reproduction of this formula in each container.

2. Detailed trade names or supplier names must be written next to each ingredient and its grade. The botanical names should be written in detail to specify the species and type of preparations like powders, extracts, essential oils, butter, etc. International Nomenclature of Cosmetic Ingredient (INCI) names are universal names for each kind of ingredient used in the production of cosmetic products. It represents the scientific name of each element. There may be several names for each ingredient, so adding the INCI name for each item can be useful in specifying the exact ingredient. For example, shea butter is the common or trade name, while its INCI name is Butyrospermum Parkii.

The trade name is also helpful to indicate how the item is commonly referred to; however, these names are not specific. Each supplier produces each ingredient differently, so you have to write down all the supplier's details to get the same product, whether you're producing it at home or giving it to a contract manufacturer. For example, an ingredient like xanthan gum is available in many different grades and viscosities. You need to be specific about the exact grade used to create your product. The same thing goes for emulsifying agents in different varieties and even vitamins containing different properties. An example of proper information about an emulsifier is Montanov 68 MB.

3. You can also include the function or element of each ingredient. This comes in handy when you want to adjust different features in your product to easily spot the functionality of each element and know which one needs to be altered. For example, beeswax is used to create a firmer texture in a face cream, so you can record this function next to the ingredient in your formula.

4. The ingredients must be written in phases and not just be listed as individual ingredients. It is important to write the method specifically depending on each material. For example, suppose you're producing a cream emulsion. In that case, there should be an aqueous phase and an emulsifying phase in addition to other ingredients. The ingredients could be divided into three phases: A, B, and C. Phase A could be the aqueous phase, including water, xanthan gum, and glycerin. Phase B could be the oily phase, including butter, oils, and emulsifiers. Phase C includes the ingredients added after the emulsion, like vitamins or preservatives.

5. When writing each step in the method part, include information about the temperature of each ingredient, like water. For example, write "add to water at 80° C"

instead of writing "add to hot water." It is important to include the speed of mixing (whether low or high-speed mixing) and not just write "stir for 10 minutes." Time is not an accurate measure here because what is enough for a small batch will not be enough for a larger one. The size of your batch and type of equipment will have different time specifications. You should also include an endpoint to know when each step is completed. This may include the shape or texture of the product after stirring. You can write, "Stir at high speed until a glossy emulsion or a homogeneous gel is formed."

6. The formula must include a final pH value of the product with a specific range to allow for changes over the years. The range should be small to ensure the quality of the product is still valid until the expiration date (e.g., 5.5 ±0.25). It shouldn't be a wide range because this indicates the product is unstable or has a lower shelf-life than you intended.

To produce a face cream, you can use a few basic elements and some essential oils depending on your skin type and the essence you prefer. The basic elements include a carrier oil like avocado or jojoba, which contains hydrating properties and retains the natural oils in the skin.

Beeswax is used to protect the skin from different weather conditions. Nut butter, like shea or coconut butter, acts as the base of the cream, contributing the most to its soft texture. The final, most common ingredient is grapefruit seed extract, which acts as an antibiotic and antifungal agent. Other common additives are vitamins, essential oils, sunscreens, and minerals.

Before choosing essential oils, you need to determine which one is best suited for your skin type. For example, citrus oils are great for oily skin, while avocado or sesame oils are better for dry skin. You can also test a sample on your skin but make sure it is diluted to avoid a severe reaction. The perfect oil for your skin should be absorbed easily without causing any rashes.

How to Calculate the Percentage of Each Ingredient

A percentage is a proper way to measure an ingredient in your formula. It is a number expressed as a part of 100, which is the total sum of a percentage. It makes the measurements clearer and the calculations easier to formulate a small batch or a large one. Industrial measurements use the metric system because it is easier to calculate percentages from grams and kilograms.

From Recipes to Formulas

The first step is to weigh each ingredient in grams. If your recipe calls for one cup of shea butter, measure one cup and weigh it in grams. Record the weight of each solid and liquid ingredient in the recipe. After weighing all the ingredients, add them up and find the total weight. Then divide each item by the total weight of the ingredients and multiply the result by 100 to find the percentages. Each component's percentage will contain fractions, so round them up to get as near to the whole sum as possible. All the percentages should add up to 100.

The next step is to decide the weight of your product. Let's assume you are producing a 250 g container. To convert the percentage to grams, consider that 1% equals 1 gram, 100% equals 100 grams, and so forth. Divide the 250 grams by 100 to get the factor you need to multiply by each ingredient's percentage. The result is 2.5. If you're going for a 500-gram container, your factor will be 5, a 300-gram container, 3, and so on.

Let's say you're using shea butter in your mixture, which you calculated to be 25% by weight according to the calculation in the previous paragraph. To calculate the number of grams needed in a 250-gram container, you should multiply 25 by 2.5, which equals 62.5 grams. This means that, in a 250-gram container, you'll use 62.5 grams of shea butter. Repeat this calculation with each ingredient to create your product. When you add the weights of all the ingredients in grams, they should add up to 250 grams.

Some elements can't exceed a certain percentage due to safety concerns, including preservatives and certain essential oils. Due to these restrictions, you may have to adjust the percentages of the rest of the ingredients that you can afford to increase or decrease without raising any safety concerns. If you had such an issue with your preservative

content, you could alter the water percentage to get your total
to 100%.

CONCLUSION

Herbal remedies have been used by many cultures for thousands of years. They are effective at treating some of the most common ailments in your life and since they can be grown in your backyard or easily accessed no matter where you are they are the perfect way to keep your body healthy.

Even the modern western world, with all its modern medications, finds that using herbal remedies can be better and safer for the whole body. In the last decades, more species of plants and ways to use them have been discovered. New medicinal plants have had their chemical composition isolated and analyzed using chemical extraction or other methods.

What we have found is that medicinal plants usually contain chemicals known as alkaloids and flavonoids that possess powerful healing properties and are a great way to get the good stuff out of the ground and into your body. Herbal medicine can help with everything from:

- Relieving muscle pain, headache, helping to heal from sprains and bone fractures

- Healing skin conditions like eczema, psoriasis, rashes or allergic reactions

- Helping with depression, anxiety, chronic fatigue, brain function and memory

- Dealing with asthma and respiratory issues

- Supporting digestion regularly, calming stomach aches, and helping with IBS, Crohn's or Colitis

- Relieving cold and flu symptoms, helping the body to heal, and general immune system support

Plants are used to cure various problems, and you may have even quit taking your prescription medications after discovering a natural substitute. The natural compounds found in certain medicinal plants play an important role in maintaining health and healing, especially when used alongside other healthcare treatments.

You can either buy or make them in the form of extracts such as tinctures, teas, salves, and other forms. Individuals can also apply the oils directly to the skin as part of a healing process.

Many people have never heard of medicinal plants and they're not familiar with the fact that plant-based medicine is a vital part of our global health system. We have written this guide to make people aware of how easy, safe, and accessible herbal medicine is.

In this guidebook, we have spent some time looking at the various herbal remedies that you may want to try out for your health. Whether you are just considering herbs for your personal use or you are curious about how this works and how much work you will need to put into using herbs, this guidebook will answer all your questions and more.

Stop being stuck using medications that eat at your budget each month, medications that don't work all that well or just mask the problem, or medications that are not that safe for the body. Instead, consider using some herbal remedies and see how much better you can make your overall health.

DID YOU ENJOY THE BOOK? WE'D LOVE TO HEAR YOUR THOUGHTS!

Thank you for purchasing & reading our book! We do have a favor to ask from you, and that's if you can leave a review on our Amazon page!

As a small, independent publishing company with a tiny marketing budget, reviews are our livelihood on this platform. Even if it's just a sentence or two, it would make all the difference and would be very much appreciated.

If you already have, we'd like to thank you so much for leaving the review!

If you haven't yet, you can simply write your review here on our page through one of these links or scan the QR Codes.

If you're from the US, you can leave a review by clicking this link or scanning the code:

SCAN ME

https://amazon.com/review/create-review?&asin=1804210239

421

If you're from the UK, you can leave a review by clicking this link or scanning the code:

SCAN ME

https://amazon.co.uk/review/create-review?&asin=1804210239

We pour our heart and soul into our books, and reviews like yours help us spread our message and get our work into the hands of more people.

We appreciate you, and we just want to say thank you.

Sincerely,

Small Footprint Press

REFERENCES AND ADDITIONAL READING

American Indian Health and Diet Project. (2022). *Foods Indigenous to the Western Hemisphere.* AIHDP. https://aihd.ku.edu/foods/

Angelfire.(2022). *Meanings and Legends of Flowers.* Angelfire.com.
https://www.angelfire.com/journal2/flowers/v.html

Encyclopedia Britannica. (2022). *Herb: Sorrel.* https://www.britannica.com/plant/sorrel

Grieve, M. (1931). *Botanical.com: A Modern Herbal.* Botanical.com. https://www.botanical.com

Indiana Medical History Museum. (2022). *Guide to the Medicinal Plant Garden.* Indiana Medical History Museum. https://www.imhm.org/resources/Documents/medicinalgardenbook[1].pdf

Lee, Robert. (2009). *The Last Drop of Living: A Minimalist's Guide to Living the High Life on a Low Budget.* Las Vegas: Createspace.

Lee, Robert. (2011). *Eating Wild.* (Revised Ed., 2019) Winnipeg: Romanie Press.

Lee, Robert. (2021). *Eating Wild.* Eating Wild Blog. https://www.eatingwild.blogspot.com

Mayo Clinic. (2022). *Integrative Medicine and Health Research Program: Herbs and Dietary Supplements Study.* Mayo Clinic Online. https://www.mayo.edu/research/centers-programs/integrative-medicine-health-research/research-studies/herbs-dietary-supplement-studies

Mother Earth Living. (2022). *Natural Remedies.* Motherearthliving.com https://www.motherearthliving.com/health-and-wellness/natural-remedies/

Mount Sinai. (2022). *Health Library Search.* Mount Sinai Organization of New York State. https://www.mountsinai.org/health-library/search

National Center for Biotechnology Information. (2022). *User Guide.* National Library of Medicine. https://www.ncbi.nlm.nih.gov/pmc/

The Naturopathic Herbalist. (2022). *Herbs by Common Name.* Thenaturopathicherbalist.com https://thenaturopathicherbalist.com/herbs-common/

Wikipedia. (2022). *Asparagus Acutifolius.* Wikipedia.org. https://en.wikipedia.org/wiki/Asparagus_acutifolius

Wikipedia. (2022). *List of food plants native to the Americas.* Wikipedia.org. https://en.wikipedia.org/wiki/List_of_food_plants_native_to_the_Americas

Wikipedia. (2022). *List of Lunar Deities*. Wikipedia.org. https://en.wikipedia.org/wiki/List_of_lunar_deities

Wonderment Gardens. (2020). *Definitions of Herbal Actions and Properties*. Wondermentgardens.com. https://wondermentgardens.com/herbal-actions-and-properties/

(2016). *Homestead Pharmacy: How to make herbal capsules*. Joybilee Farm. https://joybileefarm.com/how-to-make-herbal-capsules/

Ali Karimi, M. (2022). *Herbal versus synthetic drugs; beliefs and facts*. National Library of Medicine. https://www.ncbi.nlm.nih.gov/pmc/articles/PMC5297475/

Hayes, Allie. (2019). *People are sharing the weirdest ways they've seen someone misuse an everyday object and LOL*. Buzzfeed. https://www.buzzfeed.com/alliehayes/weird-uses-of-everyday-items-reddit

Blog.mountainroseherbs. (2017). *How to make herbal infusions & decoctions for wellness support*. Mountain Rose Herbs. https://blog.mountainroseherbs.com/herbal-infusions-and-decoctions

Booker, A. (2022). *Which is deadlier—herbal remedies or conventional medicines?* https://theconversation.com/which-is-deadlier-herbal-remedies-or-conventional-medicines-74498

Carolyn. (2019). *How to choose high quality herbs and herbal remedies - bloom institute.* The Bloom Institute Center for Herbal Education. https://bloominstitute.ca/how-to-choose-high-quality-herbs/

Chaunie Brusie. (2019). *What are the most effective natural antibiotics?* Healthline. https://www.healthline.com/health/natural-antibiotics#myrrh

Dickinson, R. (2016). *3 Types of Herbal First Aid Kits.* https://thesurvivalmom.com/3-types-herbal-first-aid-kits/

EcoWatch. (2022). *10 reasons to consider herbal medicine the next time you're not feeling well.* https://www.ecowatch.com/herbal-medicine-2009451657.html

Ekor, M. (2022). *The growing use of herbal medicines: issues relating to adverse reactions and challenges in monitoring safety.* Natural Library of Medicine. https://www.ncbi.nlm.nih.gov/pmc/articles/PMC3887317/

Morgan, Emma. (2016). *What netflix's 'broken' taught us about counterfeit cosmetics - the tease.* https://www.thetease.com/what-netflixs-broken-taught-us-about-counterfeit-cosmetics/

Gwynn, J., & Hylands, P. (2022). *Plants as a source of new medicines—Drug Discovery World (DDW).* https://www.ddw-online.com/plants-as-a-source-of-new-medicines-1045-200008/

Healthline. (2016). *I was misdiagnosed: what happens when your doctor gets it wrong.* https://www.healthline.com/health/misdiagnosis-stories

Herbalismroots. (2016). *Preparation Methods of Herbs.* https://herbalismroots.com/preparation-methods-herbs/

Justis, A. (2016). *How to make an herbal decoction.* https://theherbalacademy.com/herbal-decoction/

Maitri, Zen. (2016). *What are herbal tinctures?* https://www.zenmaitri.com/blogs/news/what-are-herbal-tinctures

Meagan. (2014). *How to test herbs for allergic reactions - growing up herbal.* https://growingupherbal.com/test-herbs-for-allergic-reactions/

Meagan. (2015). *Determining herbal dosages - growing up herbal.* https://growingupherbal.com/herbal-dosages/

Meagan. (2015). how to source quality herbs - growing up herbal. https://growingupherbal.com/source-quality-herbs/

Meagan. (2015). *Using herbs: herbal syrups, honeys, and oxymels - growing up herbal.* https://growingupherbal.com/using-herbs-herbal-syrups-honeys-and-oxymels/

Meagan. (2015). *Using herbs: herbal tinctures, glycerites, and vinegars - growing up herbal.* https://growingupherbal.com/using-herbs-herbal-tinctures-glycerites-and-vinegars/

Meagan. (2015). *Using herbs: herbal washes, compresses, and fomentations - growing up herbal.* https://growingupherbal.com/using-herbs-herbal-washes-compresses-and-fomentations/

Meagan. (2015). *Using herbs: tools of the trade - growing up herbal.* https://growingupherbal.com/herbal-tools-of-the-trade/

Meagan. (2015). *Using herbs: wildcrafting and preserving herbs - growing up herbal.* https://growingupherbal.com/wildcrafting-and-preserving-herbs/

Medicalxpress. (2017). *2 critically ill in San Francisco after drinking toxic tea.* https://medicalxpress.com/news/2017-03-critically-ill-san-francisco-toxic.html

Mossy Meadow Farm. (2016). *Herbal remedies for beginner's | how to make a decoction.* https://www.mossymeadowfarm.com/blog/herbal-remedies-for-beginners-how-to-make-a-decoction

NCCIH. (2022). *How herbs can interact with medicines.* https://www.nccih.nih.gov/health/tips/tips-how-herbs-can-interact-with-medicines

Robinett, R. (2021). *Choosing the right herbs for you, according to a herbalist | well+good.* https://www.wellandgood.com/right-herbs-for-you/

Raman, R. MS, RD. (2018) *Echinacea: benefits, uses, side effects and dosage.* https://www.healthline.com/nutrition/echinacea#benefits

St. Luke's Hospital. (2016). *Burns | complementary and alternative medicine.* https://www.stlukes-stl.com/health-content/medicine/33/000021.htm

Williams, NP. (2022). *Herbal versus synthetic medicines.* https://www.news-medical.net/health/Herbal-versus-Synthetic-Medicines.aspx

Wishgardenherbs. (2018) *Natural remedies for insect bites & stings.* https://www.wishgardenherbs.com/blogs/wishgarden/natural-remedies-insect-bites-stings

Yang, L., Hou, D., Li, Y., Hu, Z., & Zhang, Y. (2018). A network pharmacology approach to investigate the mechanisms of Si-Jun-Zi decoction in the treatment of gastric precancerous lesions. *Traditional Medicine Research,* 3(6), 273-285.